OVERCOMING HEART DISEASE

DEDICATION

I offer this book in honor of my father, Vitalis wealth and my late mother Gladys .A .Miran. My father's impactful character greatly influenced my perspectives, while my mother introduced me to patient care during my high school years, fostering a deep sense of compassion for those patient under my care.

PREFACE

Heart disease is one of the most common health conditions that affects millions of people worldwide. Whether you're dealing with high blood pressure, coronary artery disease, or any other type of cardiovascular condition, it can be overwhelming to navigate through all the information and treatments available. This book aims to provide readers with a

comprehensive guide to prevent, manage and recover from heart disease.

In this book, we will cover various aspects of heart disease including its causes, symptoms, risk factors, diagnosis and treatments. We will delve deep into lifestyle modifications such as diet changes, exercise routines, stress management techniques, and smoking cessation programs that have been proven effective in preventing heart disease.

We will also explore the latest advancements in medical technology and surgical procedures used to treat heart diseases. From minimally invasive surgeries to non-invasive interventions, we will discuss each option in detail and help readers make informed decisions about their treatment plan.

Moreover, we understand that living with heart disease can be challenging, which is why we will include practical advice on coping mechanisms and support networks. Readers will learn how to deal with emotional upheavals and physical discomfort during recovery, as well as tips for maintaining a positive mindset throughout their journey towards healing.

Finally, we will introduce complementary therapies such as acupuncture, yoga, meditation, and herbal remedies that can aid in managing heart disease. These holistic approaches can provide additional benefits beyond convention and promote overall wellness.

Overall, this book serves as a valuable resource for anyone looking to conquer heart disease. With expert guidance, practical advice, and cutting-edge research, readers will gain the knowledge they need to take control of their heart health and live a fulfilling life.

CHAPTER 1:

INTRODUCTION: IMPORTANT OF HEART HEALTH

Heart disease isn't just one health problem. It's actually made up of different issues

that work either in isolation or together to damage your heart. It can include:

Blood cholesterol: When certain types of blood cholesterol are abnormal, the

main arteries leading to the heart are more likely to become clogged.

High blood pressure: When your arteries become stiff and/or narrowed, the

pressure inside them builds, which causes blood flow to become more turbulent. End

result: The lining of the arteries is more likely to become damaged.

Heart attack: This happens when a blood clot blocks the flow of blood through

one or more of the blood vessels that feed the heart

muscle. Interrupted blood flow

to the heart can damage or destroy a part of the heart muscle.

Stroke: This is just like a heart attack, but it happens inside the brain. Arteries

leading to the brain are narrowed or blocked and too little blood reaches it, causing

some of your brain cells to die.

Heart failure: Heart failure occurs when a heart can't pump enough blood to meeta body's needs. This often happens after a heart attack, when the heart

Is too damaged to pump normally.

The human heart is a complex organ responsible for pumping oxygenated blood throughout the body, providing essential nutrients and oxygen to cells, tissues, and organs. It is crucial for our survival, as even a small malfunction can lead to severe complications. However, despite its vital role in our body, many people overlook the importance of taking care of their heart health until it's too late. In this chapter, we will explore why heart health should be a top priority and the consequences of neglecting it.

One reason why heart health is so important is

because heart disease is the leading cause of death globally. According to the World Health Organization (WHO), approximately 18 million deaths occur annually due to cardiovascular diseases, including coronary heart disease, stroke, and hypertensive heart disease. Moreover, these numbers are expected to rise as populations age and lifestyles become increasingly unhealthy.

Cardiovascular diseases can have devastating effects on individuals and communities. They not only impact physical health but also mental and social wellbeing. Living with heart disease can limit daily activities, reduce quality of life, and increase healthcare costs. Additionally, heart disease can strain family dynamics, relationships, and financial stability. Therefore, prioritizing heart health can not only improve individual outcomes but also benefit society as a whole.

Furthermore, heart disease is largely preventable with proper lifestyle choices and early detection. By making healthy dietary, exercise, and stress management habits, individuals can significantly reduce their risk of developing heart disease. Early detection and intervention can also prevent serious complications and improve outcomes. Regular checkups, screenings, and monitoring can detect abnormalities before they progress into more significant issues.

The importance of heart health cannot be overstated. Neglecting heart health can result in severe complications, decreased quality of life, increased healthcare costs, and strained social and economic systems. Prioritizing heart health through proper lifestyle choices and regular health screenings can lead to better outcomes and contribute to a healthier population.

* Heart disease is not just an issue for older adults; it can affect individuals of all ages. For example, heart attacks and strokes can occur at any time, regardless of age or other factors. This highlights the need for everyone to take responsibility for maintaining a healthy heart.

* Heart disease disproportionately affects certain groups, such as those from low-income backgrounds, people of color, and women. These disparities highlight the need for targeted interventions and education to address the unique challenges faced by these populations.

* The economic burden of heart disease is significant, both for individuals and society as a whole. According to a report by the American Heart Association, heart

disease accounts for nearly $350 billion in annual healthcare spending in the United States alone. Addressing the root causes of heart disease can help mitigate this cost and improve overall public health.

* Finally, investing in research and innovation related to heart health can yield tremendous benefits for patients and healthcare providers alike. Advances in medical technology, treatment options, and prevention strategies can save lives, improve outcomes, and reduce healthcare costs.

By emphasizing the multiple facets of the importance of heart health, readers can gain a deeper understanding of why it is a critical aspect of overall health and wellbeing.

Heart disease stands as the primary cause of death in the United States for both men and women, surpassing the combined toll of all cancer types. Roughly half of these fatalities stem from sudden cardiac death, where individuals perish shortly after symptoms emerge, often due to factors like clotting or fatal irregular heart rhythms. Left ventricular hypertrophy, a result of prolonged high blood pressure, is a common contributor. Alarmingly, a significant portion of sudden cardiac death victims, 55% of men and 68% of women, show no prior signs of substantial heart issues. This disease claims lives prematurely, often without the chance of reaching medical care. However, the nutritional regimen outlined here offers a promising shield against heart attacks and sudden cardiac death, even for those grappling with advanced heart disease. It boasts the potential to dramatically reduce cholesterol and blood pressure, and even reverse obstructive coronary artery disease (CAD), potentially eliminating the need for invasive interventions like angioplasty or bypass surgery for most individuals. Unless facing rare circumstances such as advanced valve damage, genetic anomalies, or electrical pathway disorders, most people should find it feasible to reverse any existing heart ailments. In essence, this program not only reduces cholesterol but also addresses other risk factors, including the normalization of blood pressure and the reduction of LDL cholesterol.

• Reduce and standardize your blood pressure

• Decrease your low-density lipoprotein (LDL) cholesterol.

• Decrease fasting glucose levels and address type 2 diabetes.

• Regulate bowel function to normal levels.

• Enhance immune function, reducing susceptibility to infections.

• Sustain youthful vitality as you grow older,

experiencing slower aging.

This method offers the most efficient and safest approach to reducing your blood pressure and cholesterol. Moreover, it equips you with information that greatly diminishes the likelihood of experiencing a heart attack, potentially saving lives. By improving your nutrition to lower cholesterol and blood pressure, you significantly decrease the risk of heart disease compared to relying solely on medication. Other nutritional plans, backed by clinical practice and research, have shown effectiveness in preventing and reversing heart disease, often resembling this one. However, the insights shared in this book elevate this science further. Drawing from twenty-five years of clinical experience in reversing heart disease in numerous patients through nutritional excellence, this book provides comprehensive protocols, medical guidance, and detailed application instructions not only for heart disease prevention and reversal but also for averting sudden cardiac death, stroke, and dementia. My extensive patient interactions have provided invaluable insight, enabling me to offer tailored advice to address individual needs. The knowledge acquired here will empower you to overcome barriers to dietary changes, particularly since such transitions can be challenging due to the addictive nature of unhealthy foods.

CHAPTER 2:

UNDERSTANDING THE STRUCTURE AND FUNCTION OF THE HEART

The heart is a muscular organ located in the chest cavity that pumps blood throughout the body. It consists of four chambers: two upper chambers called the atria and two lower chambers called the ventricles. The right atrium receives oxygenated blood from the body and passes it into the right ventricle, which then pumps it out to the lungs via the pulmonary artery. On the left side of the heart, deoxygenated blood from the body flows into the left atrium and then into the left ventricle, which pumps it out to the rest of the body via the aorta.

The walls of the heart chambers are lined with specialized cells called cardiomyocytes, which contract to pump blood through the heart. In addition to its role as a pump, the heart also acts as a filter, removing waste products and damaged red blood cells from circulation.

The heart plays a crucial role in regulating blood flow and supplying nutrients and oxygen to tissues throughout the body while simultaneously removing waste products. Proper maintenance of the heart, including regular exercise, healthy diet, and appropriate medication management when necessary, is essential for optimal health and wellbeing.

The heart plays several essential functions that are vital for maintaining the overall health and functioning of the body. Here are some of the most important ones:

1. Pump blood throughout the body: The main function of the heart is to pump oxygenated blood throughout the circulatory system. It accomplishes this by contracting and relaxing in a rhythmic manner called cardiac muscle contractions.

2. Regulate blood pressure: The heart pumps blood out at constant pressure, which helps regulate blood flow and maintain healthy arterial pressure levels.

3. Filter waste products: Blood carries waste products and metabolic byproducts that must be eliminated from the body. The heart works closely with the kidneys to filter these substances from the circulation and expel them via urine.

4. Supply nutrients and oxygen to organs: The heart delivers oxygenated blood to tissues and cells throughout the body, supplying them with the energy and nutrients necessary for proper functioning.

5. Control heart rate and rhythm: The autonomic

nervous system regulates heart rate and rhythm through the actions of sympathetic and parasympathetic nerves. The heart responds to signals sent by these nerves, either increasing or decreasing its activity to meet the demands of the body.

6. Support life-saving mechanisms: The heart plays a crucial role in certain emergency situations, such as cardiopulmonary resuscitation (CPR), where it helps keep oxygenation flowing to the brain and other vital organs until medical attention arrives.

7. Facilitate movement and exercise: During physical activity, the heart increases its output to supply muscles with oxygenated blood and remove waste products. This process supports muscular contraction and contributes to efficient movement.

The heart performs numerous functions that are integral to survival and health. Its unique design and specialized physiology enable it to operate with precision and adapt to changing circumstances, ensuring optimal functioning under various conditions.

For many years, it was believed that the heart functioned merely as a mechanical pump, transporting oxygen-depleted blood to the lungs where it absorbed oxygen, turning the blood red, before circulating it throughout the body. The prevailing notion was that as long as the heart received a steady supply of blood, like any other pump, it would continue to function smoothly. It was believed that maintaining clear arteries to ensure uninterrupted blood flow would sustain proper heart function.

We now understand that the heart is far more than just a pump; it functions as a miniature brain, complete with its own neurons, and produces hormones and an electrical field. Achieving optimal health requires more than just a healthy pump; it necessitates healthy neurons within the heart, as well as healthy nerves connecting it to the brain and other body parts. Additionally, the heart's cells must be healthy to contract and relax effectively, ensuring proper blood circulation throughout the body. This intricate cycle requires nutrients and co-factors to sustain. To maintain optimum heart health, it's crucial to ensure every cell in the body functions optimally. Focusing solely on heart and blood vessel health, while neglecting the rest of the body, is akin to only attending to the spark plugs in a car without changing the oil or performing other maintenance tasks; eventually, the engine will fail. Cardiologists, like other specialists, should consider more than just the cardiovascular system, recognizing the interconnectedness of all bodily systems. Holistic health approaches view the body as a network of interconnected organs, tissues, and cells influenced by various factors, including lifestyle choices and genetics. Understanding this interconnected system is crucial for promoting good health.

CHAPTER 3:

RISK FACTORS FOR HEART DISEASE

Heart disease is a leading cause of death worldwide and can be influenced by various risk factors. Including:

1. High Blood Pressure (Hypertension): Elevated blood pressure puts stress on the cardiovascular system, increasing the risk of damage to the heart and blood vessels.

2. Smoking: Nicotine constricts the blood vessels, raising blood pressure and reducing blood flow, which increases the risk of heart attack and stroke.

3. Obesity: Excess weight, especially around the waist, can lead to metabolic disorders like high blood sugar and insulin resistance, contributing to cardiovascular disease.

4. Diabetes: High glucose levels can damage blood vessels over time, weakening them and increasing the likelihood of developing heart disease.

5. Dyslipidemia: Abnormal lipid profiles, such as high triglyceride or low HDL ("good") cholesterol levels, can contribute to plaque buildup in your arteries, increasing your risk of heart attacks and strokes.

6. Family History: Having family members with a

history of heart disease may increase your chances of developing the condition due to genetic predispositions.

7. Age: As you age, your risk of heart disease generally increases. This is partly due to changes in blood vessel function, hormonal shifts, and accumulation of health conditions associated with aging.

8. Poor Diet: Consuming diets rich in saturated fats, trans fats, sodium, and added sugars can raise your risk of heart disease. In contrast, eating a diet rich in fruits, vegetables, whole grains, lean proteins, and healthy fats can help protect your heart.

9. Sedentary Lifestyle: Regular physical activity helps maintain a healthy weight, reduces inflammation, and improves circulation, all of which contribute to a lower risk of heart disease.

10. Stress: Chronic stress and mental health issues can negatively impact cardiovascular health by elevating blood pressure, releasing stress hormones, and promoting unhealthy lifestyle choices.

It's essential to understand and manage these risk factors to minimize the chance of developing heart disease. Regular checkups, a balanced diet, regular exercise, and managing any underlying health conditions can significantly reduce the risk of heart disease. Additionally, quitting smoking, limiting alcohol consumption, and addressing stress can also make a significant difference in overall heart health.

Heart disease is a complex condition that affects millions of people worldwide each year. There are many known risk factors for heart disease, including high blood pressure, high cholesterol levels, smoking, diabetes, obesity, family history of heart disease, lack of physical activity, stress, poor diet, excessive alcohol consumption, and certain medications. It's important to understand these risks in order to prevent and manage the condition effectively. If you're concerned about your own risk of heart disease, I recommend consulting with a healthcare professional who can provide personalized advice and guidance.

High blood pressure is a common condition that can lead to serious health problems if left untreated. Here are some steps you can take to lower your blood pressure naturally:

1. Eat a healthy diet: Focus on a diet rich in whole foods like fruits, vegetables, lean proteins, nuts, and seeds. These foods contain essential nutrients and antioxidants that can help lower your blood pressure levels. Avoid processed foods and those high in saturated fats, as these can increase blood pressure.

2. Exercise regularly: Regular exercise helps improve cardiovascular health, which in turn can lower your blood pressure. Aim for at least 30 minutes of moderate-intensity physical activity every day, such as walking or cycling.

3. Manage stress: Chronic stress can contribute to high blood pressure. Find ways to manage stress through relaxation techniques such as meditation, deep breathing, yoga, or tai chi.

4. Get enough sleep: Poor sleep quality can also raise blood pressure levels. Make sure you get adequate rest each night and maintain a regular sleep schedule.

5. Stay hydrated: Dehydration can cause the body to retain salt, leading to an increase in blood pressure. Make sure you drink plenty of water throughout the day to stay properly hydrated.

6. Limit alcohol intake: Excessive alcohol consumption can raise blood pressure temporarily. If you choose to drink, limit your intake to no more than one drink per day for women and two drinks per day for men.

7. Consider supplements: Certain herbs and supplements may help lower blood pressure naturally, but it is important to speak with a healthcare professional before taking any new supplements. Some examples include garlic, hawthorn berry, and omega-3 fatty acids.

It's always recommended to consult with a doctor or a nutritionist to check if this plan will be suitable for you and to make sure your health is under control while making changes to your lifestyle. Remember that managing blood pressure requires long-term effort and consistency, so it's important to stick to a healthy lifestyle consistently.

CHAPTER 4:

SYMPTOMS OF HEART DISEASE

Symptoms of heart disease can vary depending on the type of condition and how far along it has progressed. Some common symptoms include chest pain, shortness of breath, fatigue, dizziness, nausea, vomiting, sweating, weakness in the arms or legs, swelling, rapid or irregular heartbeat, difficulty sleeping at night, and feeling lightheaded when standing up quickly or lying down suddenly. These symptoms should not be ignored as they could indicate a serious underlying medical issue. If you experience any of these symptoms, seek immediate medical attention from a healthcare professional. They will perform tests such as an electrocardiogram (ECG) or echocardiogram (ECHO), which can help diagnose heart conditions and determine appropriate treatment options.

The following segment advises on symptom recognition for potential heart issues. It underscores the importance of understanding early signs, such as erectile dysfunction in men due to low testosterone levels, and fatigue, particularly in women during exertion. Additionally, it stresses the significance of addressing any unusual symptoms like chest pressure or shortness of breath promptly, as they could indicate advanced heart disease.

Heart disease is a complex condition with various symptoms that depend on its severity and location. Here are some of the most common symptoms of heart disease:

1. Chest Pain - Chest pain can be described as discomfort, pressure, tightness, or pain in the center of the chest, spreading to one or both arms, neck, jaw, or stomach.

2. Shortness of Breath - Difficulty breathing or feeling short of breath can occur with physical activity or while resting, especially if there is fluid accumulation in the lungs.

3. Fatigue - Feeling excessively tired for no apparent reason can be a symptom of heart disease, particularly if it interferes with daily activities.

4. Dizziness or Lightheadedness - Fainting or near-

fainting spells can occur, especially when changing position quickly or standing still for too long.

5. Nausea and Vomiting - In severe cases, heart disease can cause gastrointestinal distress, including nausea and vomiting.

6. Swelling - Fluid accumulation in the body, known as edema, can occur in areas such as the legs, feet, ankles, hands, face, and abdomen.

7. Rapid or Irregular Heartbeat - Abnormal heart rhythms can manifest as palpitations, skipped beats, or fluttering sensations.

8. Difficulty Sleeping - Insomnia or frequent waking during the night can be caused by heart disease, as it disrupts normal breathing patterns and causes discomfort.

9. Jaundice - Yellow skin or eyes can be a sign of heart failure, as it indicates liver damage and reduced circulation.

10. Weakness in the Arms or Legs - Reduced strength or endurance in the arms or legs can be a symptom of heart disease, especially when accompanied by shortness of breath or chest pain.

It's essential to remember that not everyone with heart disease experiences these symptoms, and some people may have non-specific symptoms like fatigue or indigestion. However, if you notice any unusual changes in your heart rate, breathing, or energy levels, it's crucial to consult a doctor immediately. Early diagnosis and treatment can save lives and improve quality of life.

Here are some specific types of heart disease:

1. Coronary artery disease (CAD): This occurs when the arteries that supply blood to the heart become narrowed due to plaque buildup. CAD can lead to angina (chest pain), myocardial infarction (heart attack), and stroke.

2. Atrial fibrillation: A disorder characterized by abnormal rhythmic contractions of the upper chamber of the heart, resulting in fast, irregular, and sometimes forceful beating of the heart.

3. Congestive heart failure (CHF): A chronic condition where the heart is unable to pump enough blood to meet the body's needs. CHF may cause symptoms such as fluid retention, shortness of breath, and edema (swelling).

4. Valvular disorders: Problems with the valves inside the heart that regulate the flow of blood between the chambers. Common valve disorders include mitral stenosis, tricuspid stenosis, and aortic stenosis.

5. Cardiomyopathy: A group of diseases that affect the structure and function of the heart muscle.

Common causes include hypertrophic cardiomyopathy, dilated cardiomyopathy, and restrictive cardiomyopathy.

6. Arrhythmogenic right ventricular cardiomyopathy: A genetic disorder of the heart muscle that primarily affects the right side of the heart. ARVC is often diagnosed through genetic testing and ECG.

7. Long QT syndrome: A rare genetic disorder of the heart that leads to abnormally slow repolarization of heart cells after each contraction. LQTS increases the risk of sudden death due to arrhythmias.

8. Pulmonary hypertension: High blood pressure in the lungs that results in increased resistance to blood flowing through the pulmonary vessels, leading to right ventricular dysfunction and potentially fatal complications.

9. Patent ductus arteriosus (PDA): A congenital defect where the ductus arteriosus, a blood vessel connecting the aorta to the pulmonary artery during fetal development, fails to close properly. PDA can result in persistent left-to-right shunting of oxygen-poor blood from the right atrium to the pulmonary artery, potentially leading to pulmonary hypertension and other health problems.

These are just a few examples of the many types of heart disease. It's important to note that not all cases of heart disease have clear symptoms, so regular checkups and monitoring with healthcare professionals can help identify potential issues early and prevent further damage. Additionally, managing lifestyle factors such as eating a healthy diet, exercising regularly, maintaining a healthy weight, avoiding tobacco products, limiting alcohol intake, and getting adequate sleep can also play a significant role in preventing heart disease.

The Secret To Whole Body Heart Health:

Unlocking the key to holistic cardiovascular wellness involves more than simply safeguarding your heart and its associated blood vessels. It necessitates prioritizing the vitality of every component within your body, from organs and tissues to cells and molecules. This sets the stage for the forthcoming chapter's argument: safeguarding every cell demands more than pharmaceuticals or medical procedures alone. Instead, embracing a heart-healthy lifestyle is paramount for comprehensive protection, ensuring longevity and sustained cardiac health for years and decades ahead. The forthcoming prescriptions outlined in this book will guide you toward achieving this goal.

CHAPTER 5 :

DIAGNOSING HEART DISEASE

Diagnosing heart disease involves a combination of medical history, physical examination, and various diagnostic tests. Here's an overview of some common methods used to diagnose heart disease:

★Medical History: Your doctor will ask about your medical history, including any family history of heart disease, any symptoms you may be experiencing (such as chest pain or shortness of breath), and other risk factors for heart disease such as high blood pressure, smoking, and diabetes.

★ Physical Examination: During the physical exam, your doctor will listen to your heartbeat, check your pulse, and perform a thorough exam of your cardiovascular system. This may include auscultation of your heart sounds, palpitation of your veins, and measurement of your blood pressure and temperature.

★ Electrocardiogram (ECG): An ECG is a noninvasive test that measures electrical activity in the heart. It helps doctors identify abnormal rhythms, conduction problems, and damage to the heart muscle.

★ Chest X-ray: A chest x-ray can help detect structural

changes in the heart and lungs, such as enlargement or calcification. However, it is not always sensitive enough to diagnose heart disease on its own.

★ Cardiac Catheterization: This invasive procedure uses a thin tube called a catheter to visualize the inside of your arteries and coronary vessels. The catheter is inserted through a small incision in your wrist or groin, and contrast dye is injected into the vessels to make them visible on fluoroscopy. This allows the doctor to assess the severity of blockages and determine if they need to be removed.

★. Magnetic Resonance Angiography (MRA): This imaging technique uses magnetic resonance technology to create detailed images of your heart and blood vessels. It is often used to evaluate patients with complex cardiac conditions and can provide information about the size, shape, and function of the heart and great vessels.

★Holter Monitoring: This is a continuous recording of electrocardiographic tracings over several hours or days. It can help detect abnormal heart rhythms, conduction disturbances, and arrhythmias that may not occur during routine testing.

★Blood Tests: Several blood tests can be used to measure markers of inflammation, lipid levels, glucose control, and liver and kidney function. These results can give clues about the underlying cause of heart disease.

★ Imaging Studies: Other imaging studies, such as echocardiography, transesophageal echocardiography (TEE), and positron emission tomography (PET) scans, can also be used to diagnose heart disease and evaluate its extent and severity.

It's important to note that these tests are just tools to aid in diagnosis, and the final diagnosis will depend on a careful interpretation of all available evidence.

Importance Of Diagnosing The Heart :

Early detection and diagnosis of heart disease is critical because timely treatment can prevent further damage to the heart and improve outcomes. Here are some benefits of diagnosing the heart:

★Improved Treatment Outcomes: When heart disease is diagnosed early, individuals can receive appropriate treatment earlier in the course of their condition. This means that treatments can be more effective at preventing further damage to the heart and improving overall health outcomes.

★Prevention of Complications: Untreated heart disease can lead to serious complications such as heart attacks, strokes, and congestive heart failure. By diagnosing heart disease early, individuals can take steps to prevent these complications from occurring.

★ Better Management of Risk Factors: Identifying and managing risk factors associated with heart disease such as high blood pressure, cholesterol, obesity, and diabetes early can significantly reduce the risk of developing additional cardiovascular diseases in the future.

★ Increased Quality of Life: Early diagnosis and management of heart disease can improve quality of life by reducing symptoms and enabling individuals to participate in activities that were previously restricted due to their heart condition.

★Reduced Healthcare Costs: Early diagnosis and treatment of heart disease can result in reduced healthcare costs by avoiding unnecessary hospitalizations and procedures and minimizing long-term complications associated with untreated heart disease.

Prompt diagnosis and treatment of heart disease is essential for achieving optimal health outcomes and reducing the burden of heart disease on individuals and society

Non-invasive Testing for Heart Disease

Non-invasive testing for heart disease refers to various diagnostic methods that do not involve surgery or insertion of devices into the body. These tests provide information about the structure and function of the heart without causing any harm to the patient. Some examples of non-invasive testing for heart disease include:

1. Echocardiography: The echocardiograph produces images of the heart using high-frequency sound waves. It is a safe and painless procedure that can be done quickly and easily. Echocardiography is commonly used to diagnose and monitor heart conditions such as valve disorders, congenital heart disease, cardiac amyloidosis, hypertensive heart disease, and chronic systolic left ventricular dysfunction.

2. Electrocardiography: An ECG captures the electrical signals generated by the heart muscle and transmitted through the chest wall to the surface electrodes. ECG is an easy and quick procedure that does not require any special preparations or training. It is useful for identifying arrhythmias, conduction disorders, QT prolongation, and ST segment elevation or depression, which are all potential indicators of heart disease.

3. Holter monitoring: Holter monitors are worn around the neck or waist for several hours or days and record electrical impulses from the heart throughout the day. They can detect subtle changes in heart rate variability and rhythm that might not be noticeable

during a resting ECG. This type of continuous monitoring allows doctors to better understand how the heart functions under normal and stressed conditions.

4. Nuclear medicine tests: These tests use radioactive tracers and imaging technology to visualize the function of the heart and isssssts blood vessels. Common nuclear medicine tests for the heart include stress tests, myocardial perfusion scans, and radionuclide angioplasties. These tests are typically performed in hospitals or specialized clinics and require careful administration and interpretation by trained professionals.

5. Stress testing: During a stress test, patients perform physical activities that increase their heart rate and blood pressure, such as walking on a treadmill or cycling. Blood samples and ECG readings are taken before, during, and after the exercise, allowing doctors to determine how well the heart is functioning under stress. Stress testing is often used to diagnose coronary artery disease and to guide treatment decisions.

6. Carotid artery ultrasound: This test involves using ultrasound to examine the blood vessels in the neck and head. Plaque buildup in these vessels can increase the risk of stroke and other heart-related problems. While the procedure is generally safe, there is a small risk of bleeding if the arteries are punctured

during the examination.

7. Transcranial Doppler study: This test uses ultrasound to measure the velocity of blood flow through the cerebral veins. It can detect signs of abnormal blood flow, such as increased turbulence or slowing down of the blood. While this test is usually considered safe, there is a slight risk of bleeding if the vessel walls are damaged during the examination.

In summary, non-invasive testing for heart disease offers a variety of valuable diagnostic tools that allow healthcare providers to assess the structure and function of the heart without putting patients at risk. Each test has its own unique advantages and limitations, and choosing the right test for a particular patient requires careful consideration of their individual needs and circumstances.

Non-invasive testing for heart disease plays a crucial role in diagnosing and monitoring cardiovascular conditions. It allows doctors to assess various aspects of the heart function without putting the patient at risk of harm. Here are some key reasons why non-invasive testing is important:

1. Early diagnosis: With non-invasive testing, healthcare providers can detect changes in the heart before symptoms become noticeable. This means that treatment can begin sooner, potentially preventing further complications.

2. Monitoring progression: Non-invasive testing can help track the progression of heart disease over time. This is particularly useful when managing chronic conditions like coronary artery disease (CAD) or heart failure.

3. Assessing response to therapy: Non-invasive testing can be used to evaluate how well the heart responds to medical treatments, including medications and lifestyle modifications.

4. Guiding interventions: The results of non-invasive testing can inform decisions about whether additional diagnostic tests or interventions, such as surgery or angioplasty, are necessary.

5. Minimizing risks: Compared to invasive tests like cardiac catheterization, non-invasive testing poses fewer risks and side effects.

6. Lower costs: Many non-invasive tests can be performed in a clinic setting, rather than requiring hospitalization, leading to lower overall costs for both the patient and healthcare system.

7. Better patient outcomes: Non-invasive testing contributes to better understanding of the underlying causes and severity of heart disease, resulting in improved care and ultimately better patient outcomes.

8. Personalized approach: Some non-invasive tests allow physicians to customize their evaluation plans

based on each individual's unique needs, enabling personalized care.

9. Enhanced communication: Non-invasive testing facilitates open dialogue between healthcare providers and patients regarding their heart health, empowering individuals with knowledge about their condition and fostering shared decision-making.

10. Advancing research: Non-invasive testing has opened new avenues of research, helping scientists understand the complex mechanisms governing cardiovascular function and allowing for novel therapies to be developed.

Non-invasive testing for heart disease plays a vital role in the diagnosis, monitoring, and management of cardiovascular conditions. Its importance extends beyond the direct benefit to patients by guiding medical professionals, driving innovation, and contributing to our overall understanding of heart health.

CHAPTER 6:

LIFESTYLE MODIFICATION FOR HEART HEALTH

Life style modifications are essential components of any comprehensive plan for maintaining good heart health. These adjustments can significantly reduce the risk of developing heart disease or manage existing conditions more effectively. Here are some key lifestyle modifications that have been shown to improve heart health:

1. Eating a healthy diet: A balanced and nutritious diet rich in fruits, vegetables, whole grains, lean proteins, and low-fat dairy products is crucial for heart health. Limit intake of saturated fats, trans fats, cholesterol, sodium, and added sugars.

2. Regular physical activity: Engaging in regular exercise, aiming for at least 150 minutes of moderate-intensity aerobic activity per week or 75 minutes of vigorous-intensity aerobic activity per week, along with muscle-strengthening exercises on two or more days per week, helps maintain optimal weight, control blood pressure, and lower the risk of developing heart disease.

3. Quitting smoking: Smoking damages your heart

and blood vessels, increasing the risk of heart disease. Quitting smoking can help slow down or reverse this damage and reduce the risk of developing heart problems.

4. Managing stress: Chronic stress can contribute to high blood pressure and elevate the risk of heart disease. Incorporate relaxation techniques like meditation, yoga, deep breathing, or engaging in hobbies you enjoy to keep stress levels under control.

5. Getting enough sleep: Lack of sleep increases the likelihood of obesity, high blood sugar, high blood pressure, and other factors that may raise your risk of heart disease. Prioritize getting 7-9 hours of quality sleep every night to promote heart health.

6. Limiting alcohol consumption: Excessive drinking can lead to high blood pressure, irregular heartbeat, and an increased risk of stroke. Men should limit themselves to no more than two drinks per day, while women should stick to one.

7. Taking medication as prescribed: If you have been prescribed medication to manage heart disease, it's critical to take it as directed. This will help control your condition and prevent potential complications.

By incorporating these lifestyle modifications into your daily routine, you can enhance your heart health and lower your risk of developing heart disease. Remember, making lasting changes takes time and effort, but the rewards far outweigh the challenges. Consult a healthcare provider if you need guidance tailored to your specific needs and circumstances.

Life style modifications are essential components of any comprehensive plan for maintaining good heart health. These adjustments can significantly reduce the risk of developing heart disease or manage existing conditions more effectively. Here are some key lifestyle modifications that have been shown to improve heart health.

Making lifestyle modifications to improve heart health involves adopting habits and behaviors that support cardiovascular health. Here are some ways you can modify your lifestyle to improve your heart health:

1. Adopt a Heart-Healthy Diet: Eating a diet rich in fiber, vitamins, minerals, and antioxidants can help protect your heart from damage. Focus on consuming plenty of fruits, vegetables, whole grains, lean protein sources, and low-fat dairy products. Limit your intake of saturated fats, trans fats, and processed foods, which can increase your risk of heart disease.

2. Engage in Regular Physical Activity: Staying active is essential for overall health and wellness. Incorporate moderate-intensity exercise (e.g., brisk walking) for at least 150 minutes per week or vigorous-intensity exercise (e.g., running) for at least

75 minutes per week, along with muscle-strengthening activities at least two days per week. This will help you maintain a healthy weight, lower your blood pressure, and boost your heart health.

3. Quit Smoking: Cigarette smoke can harm your heart and blood vessels, increasing your risk of heart disease. Smoking cessation programs, such as nicotine replacement therapy and counseling, can help you quit smoking and support your efforts to maintain a healthy heart.

4. Manage Stress: High levels of stress can negatively impact your cardiovascular health by raising your blood pressure and increasing inflammation. Develop stress-reducing strategies, such as mindfulness, meditation, deep breathing exercises, or engaging in enjoyable hobbies. Seek professional help if needed.

5. Get Enough Sleep: Lack of sleep has been linked to numerous health issues, including an increased risk of heart disease. Prioritize getting 7-9 hours of high-quality sleep each night. Establish a consistent bedtime routine and create a comfortable sleep environment to improve your ability to fall asleep and stay asleep.

6. Limit Alcohol Consumption: While moderation may be possible, excessive drinking can lead to various health concerns, including heart disease. Men should aim for no more than two drinks per day, while women

should stick to one. Avoid binge drinking and consider seeking help if you struggle with alcohol addiction.

7. Monitor Your Health: Regular checkups with your healthcare provider are important for detecting and managing potential health issues early on. Follow your doctor's recommendations for screenings, medication management, and ongoing care to ensure your heart remains healthy.

Remember, implementing these lifestyle modifications requires consistency, discipline, and patience. Start small and gradually incorporate new habits into your daily routine. With persistence and dedication, you can make significant improvements in your heart health and reduce your risk of developing heart disease. Always consult with a healthcare professional before starting any new lifestyle modifications.

Lifestyle modification plays a crucial role in maintaining optimal heart health. By making positive changes in our daily routines, we can significantly reduce the risk of developing heart diseases and promote a healthier, longer life.

Why Lifestyle Modification is Essential for Heart Health:

1. Reduces Risk Factors: Lifestyle factors like unhealthy eating habits, lack of physical activity, smoking, chronic stress, poor sleep, and excessive

alcohol consumption contribute to the development of heart diseases. By modifying these habits, individuals can decrease their exposure to these risks, ultimately reducing the likelihood of developing heart conditions.

2. Improves Cardiovascular Health: Engaging in regular physical activity, eating a balanced diet, managing stress effectively, getting enough sleep, limiting alcohol consumption, and quitting smoking all have direct impacts on cardiovascular health. These actions can enhance the function of the heart, lower blood pressure, reduce inflammation, and improve cholesterol levels.

3. Promotes Weight Management: A healthy lifestyle often includes maintaining a healthy body mass index (BMI). Excessive weight can put additional strain on the heart, increasing the risk of heart disease. By focusing on a balanced diet, regular physical activity, and weight control measures, people can keep their hearts in good shape.

4. Supports Long-Term Well-being: Implementing a heart-friendly lifestyle not only reduces the immediate risk of heart diseases but also promotes long-term well-being. Individuals who adopt these habits tend to experience improved mental health, better cognitive functioning, enhanced energy levels, and increased longevity.

5. Encourages Prevention: Many heart diseases are preventable through lifestyle interventions. By taking proactive steps to manage their cardiovascular health, people can avoid the need for costly medical treatments, hospitalizations, and other complications associated with heart disease.

Lifestyle modifications play a vital role in promoting heart health and preventing heart diseases. Embracing these positive changes can significantly reduce the risk of developing cardiovascular problems and enhance overall quality of life. It's important to remember that even small adjustments can yield substantial benefits over time, so start today and take the first step towards a healthier heart.

CHAPTER 6:

DIET AND FRUITS RECIPES FOR HEART HEALTH

A special diet designed for heart health typically focuses on incorporating nutrient-dense foods while avoiding or limiting certain types of food known to negatively impact cardiovascular health. Here are some recommendations for creating a heart-friendly diet:

1. Eat plenty of fruits, vegetables, whole grains, lean proteins, and low-fat dairy products. These foods provide essential vitamins, minerals, fiber,

antioxidants, and phytochemicals that support heart health and help maintain optimal blood pressure, lipid profiles, and glucose levels.

2. Choose unsaturated fats from sources such as olive oil, avocados, nuts, seeds, fish, and fatty fish like salmon. Unsaturated fats can help lower bad cholesterol (LDL) levels and raise "good" HDL cholesterol levels, which contributes to a healthier heart.

3. Opt for plant sterols and stanols found in fortified margarines, spreads, and supplements. These natural substances can help block the absorption of dietary cholesterol, thereby lowering cholesterol levels in your blood.

4. Limit intake of saturated and trans fats, usually found in processed and fried foods. High consumption of these fats can increase harmful LDL cholesterol levels and lead to plaque buildup within artery walls, eventually contributing to heart disease.

5. Manage portion sizes and practice mindful eating. Overeating, especially consuming high-calorie, high-sugar, and high-sodium foods, can lead to weight gain, increased blood pressure, and higher risk of cardiovascular disease.

6. Stay hydrated by drinking adequate water and other low or zero calorie beverages like green tea or herbal teas. Dehydration can cause fluid retention, elevate

blood pressure, and contribute to the development of heart disease.

7. Avoid excessive salt and added sugars in your diet. High sodium intake can increase blood pressure and worsen existing heart conditions, while excessive sugar consumption can lead to metabolic syndrome and type 2 diabetes, both of which are linked to an increased risk of heart disease.

8. Consider adopting a Mediterranean diet pattern, characterized by generous amounts of fruits, vegetables, whole grains, legumes, nuts, and seeds; moderate amounts of fish, poultry, eggs, cheese, and yogurt; and limited red meat, processed foods, and sweets. Numerous studies suggest that this dietary approach can help lower the risk of heart disease due to its emphasis on heart-healthy nutrients and limited intake of potentially harmful substances.

9. If you have specific dietary needs or restrictions, consult with a healthcare professional or registered dietitian to ensure you receive proper guidance and nutrition support tailored to your individual situation.

Remember, it's not about cutting out your favorite foods entirely, but rather finding ways to incorporate them into a balanced diet while minimizing their potential negative effects on heart health. Consistency and moderation are key when implementing a heart-friendly diet, so make gradual changes and enjoy a variety of delicious, nutritious foods to keep your heart healthy.

Consuming fruits as part of a balanced diet can provide various vitamins, minerals, fiber, and antioxidants beneficial for heart health. Here are some fruit recommendations and recipes to consider incorporating into your daily meals.

Comsume Leafy greens to lower blood pressure

Nitrates, a type of medication used for treating chest pain (angina), function by widening the blood vessels, thereby facilitating the flow of oxygen-rich blood to the heart. Fast-acting forms of nitrates are typically administered by dissolving them under the tongue or spraying them into the mouth, resulting in nearly immediate effects. Many individuals experience relief from chest pressure or shortness of breath within five minutes of administration.

Interestingly, certain foods contain a compound similar to the active ingredient in prescription nitrates and offer comparable effectiveness, although they are not intended to replace medications. Arugula, lettuce, rhubarb, beets, pine nuts, kale, bok choy, cabbage, fennel, and spinach are examples of foods rich in nitrates, which they absorb from the soil. Upon consumption, enzymes and bacteria in the mouth, particularly in the grooves on the tongue, convert these dietary nitrates into nitrite.

1. Apples: Apples are rich in soluble fiber, which can help lower cholesterol levels and reduce the risk of heart disease. Aim for at least two medium-sized apples per day.

2. Berries: Berries such as blueberries, strawberries, and raspberries are loaded with antioxidants that protect against cell damage and inflammation, reducing the risk of heart disease. Enjoy them fresh or frozen, ideally two servings per week.

3. Avocados: Although often considered a vegetable, avocados contain monounsaturated fats that improve blood flow, lower cholesterol, and support heart health. Incorporate half an avocado per day into salads, sandwiches, or smoothies.

4. Oranges: Rich in vitamin C and potassium, oranges can help lower blood pressure and improve artery health. Aim for one medium-sized orange per day.

5. Bananas: Bananas offer natural sources of potassium and magnesium, promoting heart health by supporting blood pressure regulation and muscle relaxation. Eat one banana per day.

Recipes featuring these fruits:

1. Apple slices with peanut butter and honey: Slice an

apple into wedges, spread peanut butter onto each slice, and drizzle with honey. This quick snack provides fiber from the apple, protein and healthy fats from the peanut butter, and antioxidants from the honey.

2. Blueberry and spinach salad: Toss mixed greens with fresh blueberries, chopped walnuts, and crumbled goat cheese. Dress with balsamic vinaigrette for a refreshing lunch or dinner side dish.

3. Strawberry and avocado toast: Spread mashed avocado on a slice of whole wheat bread and top with fresh strawberries. Sprinkle black pepper and lemon juice over the avocado for added flavor and nutrition.

4. Orange and banana smoothie: Blend together one medium-sized orange, one banana, unsweetened almond milk, and a scoop of vanilla protein powder for a filling breakfast or post-workout drink.

5. Raspberry oatmeal: Cook rolled oats according to package instructions and stir in fresh raspberries during the last few minutes of cooking. Top with chopped nuts and a dollop of Greek yogurt for a satisfying breakfast or dessert.

Fruits are not only delicious but also packed with essential nutrients that contribute positively to cardiovascular health. By regularly including a variety of fruits in your diet, you can maintain optimal heart function and reduce your risk of developing heart diseases. Let's delve deeper into why certain fruits are particularly good for heart health and how you can incorporate them into your meals.

Apples are known for their high soluble fiber content, which helps lower cholesterol levels by binding to cholesterol particles and removing them from the body through stool. Additionally, eating apples has been linked to improved gut health, reduced inflammation, and a decreased risk of stroke. Two medium-sized apples per day is a reasonable recommendation, as they offer enough fiber to support heart health without causing excessive bloating. Consider adding sliced apples to your oatmeal, yogurt, or sandwich for a tasty and nutritious boost.

Berries like blueberries, strawberries, and raspberries are brimming with antioxidants that protect cells from oxidative stress caused by free radicals. These powerful compounds can cause damage to your heart tissue and contribute to the development of chronic conditions like atherosclerosis (hardening of arteries). Including berries in your meals twice a week can provide adequate antioxidant protection while minimizing the risk of overshooting recommended sugar intakes. Fresh berries make for a great snack, or you can add them to smoothies, salads, or oatmeal for added sweetness and nutrition.

Avocados might surprise you as a heart-healthy fruit choice due to their higher fat content. However, avocados primarily contain monounsaturated fats, which increase HDL (good) cholesterol levels and promote healthy blood vessel functioning. Moreover, avocados are rich in fiber, potassium, vitamin K, and folate, all of which contribute to maintaining proper heart health. Half an avocado per day should suffice, allowing you to enjoy its creaminess in salads, sandwiches, smoothies, or even on toast.

Oranges are another excellent fruit option for those looking to boost their heart health. They are packed with vitamin C, which supports collagen production and contributes to healthy skin, bones, and connective tissues. Furthermore, oranges contain potassium, which regulates blood pressure and promotes normal heart rhythm. One medium-sized orange per day provides ample amounts of these important nutrients. Squeeze fresh orange juice into your water for a burst of flavor and additional vitamin C, or include sections in salads or as a garnish for dishes.

Lastly, bananas are a convenient source of potassium and magnesium, both of which support heart health by regulating blood pressure and relaxing muscles. Eating one banana per day ensures you receive sufficient amounts of these minerals while providing a natural energy boost. Add bananas to smoothies, oatmeal, or as a topping for cereal bowls for a simple yet effective way to integrate this nutrient-dense fruit into your routine.

Incorporating a diverse selection of fruits into your diet is crucial for maintaining heart health and overall wellbeing. Choose fruits that are naturally rich in nutrients such as fiber, antioxidants, vitamins, and minerals, and aim for moderate consumption to ensure you reap the most benefits without exceeding recommended caloric intakes. Remember to consult with a healthcare professional or a registered dietitian if you need personalized advice regarding your dietary needs and goals.

Have in mind that portion control and balance are key when incorporating these fruits into your diet. While they offer numerous health benefits, consuming too many may lead to excess calorie intake and potential weight gain. Consult a registered dietitian if you have specific concerns about your dietary needs and preferences.

Following a special diet designed for heart health can bring numerous benefits,

1. Lowered risk of developing cardiovascular diseases: By incorporating heart-healthy foods and avoiding or limiting unhealthy ones, you reduce your chances of getting heart disease, stroke, and peripheral artery disease.

2. Improved cholesterol profile: A heart-friendly diet helps maintain healthy cholesterol levels, reducing your likelihood of experiencing issues like coronary heart disease and stroke.

3. Better control over blood sugar levels: Focusing on whole grains, fruits, vegetables, lean proteins, and low -fat dairy products helps regulate insulin resistance and glucose tolerance, decreasing the risk of type 2 diabetes.

4. Enhanced blood pressure management: The combination of reduced salt intake, increased potassium consumption, and regular physical activity supports maintaining optimal blood pressure levels, further benefiting heart health.

5. Weight loss and maintenance: A heart-healthy diet often involves choosing lighter, more nutrient-dense foods, which may result in weight reduction or better weight management. This is particularly important since obesity can significantly increase the risk of cardiovascular diseases.

6. Reduced inflammation: Certain foods and ingredients included in a heart-friendly diet, such as

omega-3 fatty acids, antioxidants, and polyphenols, have anti-inflammatory properties. Chronic inflammation has been associated with various health problems, including heart disease.

7. Improved overall mental and cognitive function: Some research suggests that following a Mediterranean-style diet, similar to a heart-healthy diet, may promote brain health and protect against age-related cognitive decline.

8. Increased energy and vitality: Consuming a wide range of nutrient-rich foods encourages a balanced intake of macronutrients and micronutrients, supporting energy production and overall bodily functioning.

By following a special diet designed for heart health, you can enhance your quality of life, reduce your risk of chronic diseases, and improve your overall well-being. Remember that consistency is crucial, and making small yet significant changes to your daily meals can make all the difference in promoting heart health.

Consume plant-based foods that support heart health, particularly organic ones, to foster the growth of beneficial bacteria. These bacteria produce substances that reduce inflammation, counteract toxins, and provide nourishment to cells and tissues. Conversely, consuming foods that are detrimental to heart health, such as those high in chemicals, sugars, and toxins, promotes the proliferation of harmful bacteria. These harmful bacteria produce toxins, including endotoxin, which the immune system recognizes as harmful, leading to increased inflammation when it enters the bloodstream.

Research conducted by British scientists revealed that certain foods, especially animal products, contain significant levels of endotoxin, contributing to inflammatory responses in the body. Interestingly, methods such as cooking, boiling, or acid treatment do not eliminate the inflammatory potential of these foods.

As we progress through the digestive process and into the bloodstream, the body endeavors to maintain stable glucose levels.

Not adhering to a necessary diet while dealing with a heart condition can lead to several negative consequences, including:

1. Increased risk of complications: When individuals with heart disease do not follow a proper diet, they expose themselves to higher risks of severe health conditions. For example, consuming high-sodium, high-cholesterol foods can cause blood vessels to

narrow, increasing the probability of having another heart attack or stroke.

2. Worsening symptoms: An improper diet can exacerbate existing symptoms of heart disease. For instance, eating saturated fats might trigger chest pain, shortness of breath, or irregular heartbeat in patients with angina pectoris (chest pain).

3. Slower recovery time: Proper nutrition plays a crucial role in healing after surgery or other medical procedures related to heart disease. If patients don't consume enough essential nutrients during their recovery process, it could slow down their healing time and leave them vulnerable to infections.

4. Decreased effectiveness of medication: Medications used to treat heart disease work best when combined with a healthy diet. Neglecting to eat right can decrease the efficacy of these drugs and limit their ability to manage symptoms effectively.

5. Higher healthcare costs: Poor diet choices can increase the likelihood of additional hospitalizations, surgeries, and treatments, ultimately leading to higher healthcare expenses compared to those who adhere to a recommended diet.

It is essential to understand the importance of maintaining a heart-healthy diet when dealing with heart disease. Patients should consult their healthcare providers about specific diet recommendations tailored to their individual needs and circumstances. Adherence to a proper diet, along with appropriate exercise and regular checkups, can help manage heart disease and minimize its impact on one's overall health and well-being.

CHAPTER 7

ENGAGING IN EXERCISE:

Engaging in regular physical activity is vital for maintaining a healthy cardiovascular system. Heart disease prevention and rehabilitation exercises can be an essential aspect of maintaining cardiovascular health and managing conditions associated with heart disease. Some recommended exercises for heart disease patients may include:

1. Aerobic exercise: Aerobic exercises help improve cardiovascular endurance and overall fitness levels. Activities like walking, jogging, cycling, swimming, or using a stationary bike are great options for heart disease patients. Start gradually and progress as tolerated, ideally aiming for at least 150 minutes of moderate aerobic activity per week.

2. Resistance training: Incorporate resistance training into your workout routine to build muscle strength and boost metabolism. Exercises like squats, lunges, push-ups, pull-ups, or weightlifting can help maintain bone density, reduce falls risk, and enhance functional ability in heart disease patients. Perform two to three sessions per week, focusing on all major muscle groups.

3. Flexibility and balance exercises: Improving flexibility and balance can help prevent falls and reduce the risk of injury. Yoga, tai chi, Pilates, or simple stretching routines targeting key joints and muscles can be beneficial for heart disease patients. Practice these activities one to two times per week.

4. Low-impact impact exercises: High-intensity interval training (HIIT) and plyometric exercises are not suitable for everyone, especially those with certain types of heart disease. Instead, opt for low-impact alternatives like step aerobics, water aerobics, or dancing. These exercises provide similar benefits while minimizing stress on joints and reducing the risk of injury.

5. Cardiac rehabilitation programs: Participating in structured cardiac rehabilitation programs can guide heart disease patients through safe and effective exercise plans tailored to their specific condition and needs. These programs typically involve supervised workouts, education on healthy lifestyle changes, and ongoing monitoring of progress.

Remember that before starting any new exercise program, consult with your healthcare provider or a certified exercise professional to determine which activities are appropriate for your individual circumstances and goals. Gradually increase intensity and duration as your body adapts to the exercise routine, always prioritizing safety and proper form.

Regular check-ins with your healthcare team can also help monitor progress, adjust the exercise plan as needed, and address any potential concerns.

6. Rowing: This full-body exercise targets multiple muscle groups while also improving cardiovascular health.

7. Strength training: Incorporating resistance exercises into your routine can build muscular strength, which helps maintain a healthy weight, reduces strain on joints, and supports heart function.

8. Tai chi: A gentle, flowing martial art that combines stretching and relaxation, helping improve balance, flexibility, and cardiovascular health.

9. Pilates: A focused form of exercise that emphasizes core stability, coordination, and functional movements, all of which contribute to better heart health.

Remember that before starting any new exercise program, consult with your healthcare provider or a certified exercise professional to determine which activities are appropriate for your individual circumstances and goals. Gradually increase intensity and duration as your body adapts to the exercise routine, always prioritizing safety and proper form. Regular check-ins with your healthcare team can also help monitor progress, adjust the exercise plan as needed, and address any potential concerns.

Consistency is key when incorporating any exercise into your routine. Start slowly and gradually increase both duration and intensity as you become more comfortable with the chosenactivities. Always consult a healthcare professional before starting any new exercise regimen,

especially if you have pre-existing health concerns.

Engaging in regular physical activity has numerous benefits for heart health. Here are some of the most important advantages:

1. Reduced risk of coronary heart disease: Studies have shown that exercising regularly can lower the risk of developing heart disease by strengthening the heart and blood vessels, improving circulation, and helping maintain a healthy weight.

2. Lowered blood pressure: Physical activity helps regulate blood flow and blood vessel dilation, leading to reduced blood pressure. This effect is particularly significant for individuals with high blood pressure or prehypertension.

3. Better cholesterol management: Exercise can help decrease bad (LDL) cholesterol levels while increasing good (HDL) cholesterol levels. This can contribute to a healthier lipid profile and reduced risk of cardiovascular disease.

4. Enhanced circulation and oxygen delivery: Regular exercise improves blood flow and oxygen transport throughout the body, ensuring better delivery of nutrients and energy to cells and tissues.

5. Weight control: Combining regular exercise with a balanced diet can aid in achieving and maintaining a healthy weight, decreasing the risk of obesity-related heart diseases.

6. Stress reduction: Exercise releases feel-good hormones called endorphins, which can help alleviate stress and anxiety. Managing stress effectively is crucial for maintaining optimal cardiovascular health.

7. Improved mental function: Physical activity stimulates brain activity and promotes the growth of new neural connections, potentially enhancing memory, focus, and cognitive performance.

8. Increased longevity: Regular exercise has been linked to a longer lifespan, primarily due to its positive effects on heart health and overall well-being.

9. Better sleep quality: Engaging in regular physical activity can promote deeper, more restful sleep, contributing to improved overall health and well-being.

It's important to remember that engaging in regular exercise is just one component of a comprehensive approach to maintaining heart health. Proper nutrition, adequate rest, smoking cessation, and regular medical check-ups are also essential elements of a successful heart health strategy. Always consult with a healthcare professional before beginning a new exercise regimen to ensure it aligns with your individual needs and circumstances.

CHAPTER 8

Emotional health plays a significant role in shaping our physical health, including heart health. Studies have shown that chronic stress, anxiety, depression, and other mental health conditions can negatively impact cardiovascular outcomes. In fact, poor emotional health increases the risk of coronary heart disease, hypertension (high blood pressure), arrhythmias (irregular heartbeats), and heart failure. Here's how emotional health impacts the heart:

1. Chronic Stress: Long-term exposure to stress activates the sympathetic nervous system, leading to increased cortisol (stress hormone) production. This prolonged elevation of cortisol can harm blood vessels, lead to high blood pressure, and weaken the heart muscle, ultimately contributing to cardiovascular issues. Managing stress effectively through relaxation techniques, exercise, therapy, or meditation can help reduce the negative effects on heart health.

2. Anxiety Disorders: Individuals with anxiety disorders often experience rapid heart rates,

palpitations, chest pain, and shortness of breath due to heightened autonomic activity. Over time, these symptoms can lead to heart problems such as angina pectoris (chest pain) and heart attacks. Seeking treatment and practicing coping mechanisms can alleviate anxiety symptoms and improve heart health.

3. Depression: Depression has been associated with a range of cardiovascular problems, including coronary heart disease, hypertension, heart failure, and sudden death syndrome (also known as " Sudden Cardiac Death Syndrome"). The underlying causes of depression, such as sleep disturbances, low self-esteem, and social isolation, may contribute directly to these cardiovascular issues. Addressing depression through appropriate medical treatment, lifestyle changes, and social support can improve both emotional and physical well-being.

4. Anger Management: Uncontrolled anger can trigger the release of adrenaline and cortisol, which can raise blood pressure and strain the cardiovascular system over time. Learning effective ways to manage anger, such as cognitive-behavioral therapy or mindfulness practices, can help mitigate these harmful effects on the heart.

Maintaining good emotional health is just as critical for heart health as consuming a balanced diet and engaging in regular physical activity. If you suspect that your emotions may be affecting your heart health, consider seeking guidance from a healthcare provider, psychologist, or counselor who specializes in treating co-occurring mental and physical health concerns. Remember, prioritizing both emotional and physical well-being is essential for achieving and maintaining optimal health.

How Positive Emotions Can Heal:

Positive emotions act as a soothing remedy, erasing the impacts of stress and guiding us towards vitality and overall well-being.

We now understand that our hearts, along with our guts, function as miniature brains, housing their own supply of neurons that communicate with the brain. The heart can release substances that promote the release of oxytocin, known as the love hormone, which enhances our well-being and fosters connections with others. Physical actions like long hugs can trigger the release of oxytocin and improve heart health. Our emotions also impact the heart's activity; arousal from passion or anger can increase heart rate, while calmness slows it down. While it may seem challenging to simply tell ourselves to feel happy, we have some control over our emotions. Positive habits and activities such as meditation, proper breathing, and sleep significantly influence our emotional well-being. Even seemingly trivial things like human touch, interactions with pets, or treatments like acupuncture can profoundly affect mood, sleep quality, and relaxation. Remarkably, it only takes a short time, sometimes just five minutes, to experience noticeable improvements in how we feel.

Ensure to Laugh at Least Once daily.

What about a hearty laugh? Can laughter, giggles, and a playful attitude truly benefit the heart? Absolutely. Researchers found that while people watching a stressful movie like "Saving Private Ryan" experienced a 35 percent decrease in blood flow, those enjoying comedy like "Saturday Night Live" had a 22 percent increase in circulation. This boost in blood flow rivals the effects of certain prescription medications, and there are no accompanying side effects.

Set a goal to laugh daily, drawing inspiration from these suggestions:

- Opt for comedies over tragedies when choosing what to watch.

- Find opportunities to laugh at yourself instead of getting angry with yourself or others.

- Share funny stories or jokes with family members, taking turns to lighten the mood.

How Negativity Effects your heart:

Negative thoughts and feelings can break our hearts in more ways than one. Here are some ways negativity can affect the heart emotionally and physically:

1. Increased Stress Levels: Negative thinking often triggers the release of stress hormones like cortisol, which can increase the heart rate and blood pressure. Prolonged exposure to these stressors can lead to an imbalance between the body's fight-or-flight response and its rest-and-digest functions, resulting in a weakened heart.

2. Heartbreak: Experiencing a broken relationship or significant life change can cause intense emotional distress, which can manifest as physical discomfort in the heart region. This condition, known as Broken Heart Syndrome, can result in symptoms similar to those of a myocardial infarction (heart attack). Although it's not a true heart attack, it's crucial to recognize this feeling as a sign of potential emotional turmoil that could potentially exacerbate existing it heart conditions.

3. Reduced Blood Flow: Positive emotions can dilate blood vessels, allowing blood to flow freely throughout the body. On the other hand, negative emotions can constrict blood vessels, reducing blood

flow and oxygen delivery to organs, including the heart. This reduced circulation can lead to fatigue, weakness, and even cardiovascular events in severe cases.

4. Sleep Disturbances: Chronic negative thinking and emotions can interfere with quality sleep, causing insomnia and other sleep disorders. Poor sleep can disrupt the balance of hormones responsible for regulating mood and stress responses, further exacerbating any pre-existing heart conditions.

5. Increased Risk of Cardiovascular Disease: Numerous studies suggest that people who regularly experience negative emotions are at higher risk for developing cardiovascular diseases, including heart attacks and strokes. This association may be linked to factors such as increased stress levels, inflammation, and unhealthy eating habits.

6. Decreased Quality of Life: Living with constant negativity can significantly decrease overall quality of life, leading to social isolation, decreased motivation, and reduced engagement in activities that promote physical and mental well-being. A lack of enjoyment in daily life can indirectly contribute to heart health issues.

To protect your heart from the negative effects of emotions, it's important to cultivate positive attitudes, engage in healthy coping mechanisms, maintain strong relationships, and seek professional help if needed. By focusing on nurturing your emotional well-being, you'll likely see improvements in your heart health and overall well-being.

Knowing as much as you can

There exist at least two distinct groups of patients: those who conduct research prior to their appointments and those who do not. Patients in the former category typically achieve better outcomes, often because they pose more informed questions. Rather than accepting answers at face value, they are adept at following up with inquiries such as, "I came across this treatment option. Do you believe it could be beneficial for me?" Frequently, the response is affirmative. In this book, I have endeavored to undertake much of this preparatory work on your behalf. In the preceding chapter, you were introduced to recommended tests. In Part Two, numerous lifestyle recommendations are provided. However, I advise you to engage in further reading whenever possible. Within the book's appendix, numerous resources are listed. I encourage you to reference them frequently. Doing so will empower you to advocate more effectively for your health.

CHAPTER 9

MEDICAL THERAPY FOR HEART DISEASE

Medical therapies for heart disease include both pharmacological treatments (drug therapy) and non-pharmacological treatments (procedural therapy). The specific treatment approach will depend on various factors, including the type and stage of heart disease, the patient's age, medical history, and overall health status.

Drug therapy is often used to treat heart diseases caused by blockages in the coronary arteries, heart failure, and arrhythmias (irregular heartbeats). Examples of drugs used to treat heart disease include statins for reducing cholesterol levels, beta-blockers for managing hypertension and controlling heart rate, angiotensin converting enzyme inhibitors (ACEIs) and angiotensin receptor blockers (ARBs) for treating hypertension, and antiplatelet medications for preventing blood clots.

Non-pharmacological treatments, also known as procedural therapy, involve invasive procedures performed by a healthcare provider. These include coronary angioplasty and stent placement for treating blockages in the coronary arteries, pacemaker implantation for treating bradycardia (slow heartbeat), defibrillator implantation for treating ventricular fibrillation (life-threatening irregular heart rhythm), and surgical repair or replacement of damaged or diseased heart valves.

In addition to medication and procedure, lifestyle modifications such as eating a healthy diet, exercising regularly, quitting smoking, managing weight, and limiting alcohol consumption can also play a significant role in the prevention and management of heart disease.

It's important to note that every individual case of heart disease is unique, and treatment plans vary depending on the diagnosis. A healthcare provider will work closely with patients to develop personalized treatment plans that take into account their medical history, current health status, and lifestyle habits.

Medical therapies for heart disease are designed to alleviate symptoms, improve cardiovascular function, and prevent complications associated with heart disease. There are two primary types of medical therapies: drug therapy and non-pharmacological therapy. Drug therapy involves taking medications to manage heart conditions, while non-pharmacological therapy typically involves undergoing invasive procedures to address underlying issues. Here are some examples of each type of therapy:

1. Statins - these drugs reduce the level of bad

cholesterol (LDL) in the body, which helps to prevent plaque buildup in the artery walls.

2. Beta-blockers - these drugs help regulate blood pressure, slow down the heart rate, and decrease the risk of heart attacks and strokes.

3. Angiotensin Converting Enzyme Inhibitors (ACEIs) and Angiotensin Receptor Blockers (ARBs) - these drugs relax blood vessels, lower blood pressure, and reduce the risk of heart failure and stroke.

4. Antiarrhythmics - these drugs control abnormal heart rhythms and can prevent fatal arrhythmias like ventricular tachycardia and ventricular fibrillation.

5. Anticoagulants - these drugs prevent blood clots from forming and can be used to treat atrial fibrillation, pulmonary embolism, and deep vein thrombosis.

6. Diuretics - these drugs remove excess fluid from the body and can be used to treat high blood pressure and heart failure.

7. Nitrates - these drugs dilate blood vessels, reduce blood pressure, and improve oxygen delivery to the heart.

Non-Pharmacological Therapy:

1. Coronary Artery Bypass Surgery (CABG) - this surgery creates new pathways around blocked coronary arteries to restore blood flow to the heart.

2. Heart Valve Repair or Replacement - this procedure replaces or repairs damaged heart valves to improve cardiac function and prevent further damage.

3. Cardiac Catheterization - this minimally invasive procedure uses a catheter to diagnose and treat heart conditions by opening up blocked arteries or placing stents.

4. Electrocardioversion (ECV) - this procedure uses electric shocks to correct life-threatening irregular heart rhythms like ventricular fibrillation and ventricular tachycardia.

5. Pacemakers - these devices deliver electrical impulses to the heart to maintain a normal heart rate and rhythm in people with bradycardia.

6. Defibrillators - these devices deliver an electrical shock to stop dangerous heart rhythms and restore normal heart function.

In conclusion, medical therapies for heart disease are critical for maintaining optimal cardiovascular health and preventing complications related to heart disease.

While there is no one-size-fits-all solution, healthcare providers work closely with individuals to determine the best course of action based on their medical history, current condition, and lifestyle factors.

CHAPTER 10

SURGICAL TREATMENT FOR HEART DISEASE

Certainly! Surgical treatment for heart disease involves various procedures whereby surgeons operate on the heart and surrounding structures to correct or replace damaged or malfunctioning parts. Here are some common surgical treatments for heart disease:

★ Coronary Artery By Pass Grafting (CABG): This procedure is done when the coronary arteries that supply blood to the heart muscle become blocked, leading to angina or chest pain. During CABG, surgeons make small incisions in the chest, separate the ribcage, and then perform a bypass using either the patient's own blood vessels or synthetic material. The purpose of this operation is to restore normal blood flow to the heart muscle.

★Valvular Surgery: The heart has four valves that regulate blood flow within it. When these valves become dysfunctional or worn out, they may need to be repaired or replaced through valvular surgery. There are several techniques used in this procedure, including balloon dilatation, which uses a catheter to expand the narrowed valve, and open heart surgery, which involves opening up the chest cavity to access and fix the valve.

★Congenital Heart Disease Surgery: This type of surgery is mainly performed on infants and young children born with genetic heart defects. Common congenital heart disorders that require surgery include tetralogy of Fallot, truncus arteriosus, ventricular septal defect, and pulmonary atrioventricular septal defect. In these cases, surgeons may need to remove parts of the heart and connect them differently or even replace the heart entirely.

★Atrial Fibrillation Ablation: Atrial fibrillation is a common irregular heart rhythm that increases the risk of stroke and other complications. While medications can manage the condition, ablation therapy offers an alternative option. During this procedure, doctors use radiofrequency energy to destroy tiny areas of tissue inside the heart that cause arrhythmias. This helps reset the heart's electrical system and restore normal beating patterns.

★Cardiac Catheterization: This minimally invasive procedure involves threading a thin tube called a catheter through the blood vessels to reach the heart. Once inside, the doctor can diagnose problems such as blockages, plaque buildup, or leaks in the heart walls. Depending on what's found during the procedure, the doctor may recommend further testing or treatment such as stent placement or angioplasty.

Surgical treatment for heart disease can offer significant benefits for those who suffer from serious or debilitating heart conditions. As with any medical procedure, it's essential to weigh the potential risks and benefits and seek professional advice before making a decision. It's always advisable to work closely with your healthcare team to develop a personalized plan of care that considers your unique needs and circumstances.

More additional details about surgical treatment for heart disease:

★Minimally Invasive Heart Surgery: With advances in technology, many heart surgeries are now being performed using less invasive methods. These procedures involve smaller incisions, reduced trauma to the body, and faster recovery times compared to traditional open heart surgery. Examples of minimally invasive heart surgeries include robotic-assisted cardiac surgery, which allows surgeons to remotely control instruments inside the patient's body, and transcatheter aortic valve replacement (TAVR), where a new artificial valve is inserted through a small incision in the groin area.

★ Mitral Valve Repair/Replacement: The mitral valve controls the flow of blood from the left atrium into the left ventricle. If the mitral valve becomes damaged or diseased, it may not close properly, allowing blood to leak back into the atrium and increasing the risk of infection and heart failure. Surgeons can repair or replace the mitral valve during open heart surgery, often using a technique called chordaectomy, which removes excess tissue between the chords of the valve and reduces its size.

★Off-Pump Heart Surgery: Traditional heart surgery typically requires the patient's heart to stop beating temporarily while the surgeon operates on it. However, off-pump heart surgery involves keeping the heart beating continuously throughout the procedure, reducing the need for a heart-lung machine. This technique is generally reserved for patients with complex heart conditions or those at higher risk for complications associated with conventional heart surgery.

It's important to note that not all heart conditions can

be treated with surgery, and some patients may require medical management instead. Your healthcare provider will evaluate your individual case and determine the best course of action based on factors such as the severity of your symptoms, overall health status, and age. Additionally, if you do decide to undergo heart surgery, it's crucial to follow your postoperative instructions carefully and attend all scheduled appointments with your healthcare team to ensure proper healing and long-term success.

Is heart surgery the best treatment for heart disease?

heart surgery is not always the best treatment for heart disease. It depends on various factors such as the specific condition, severity of symptoms, overall health status, and age. Some heart conditions can be managed medically without requiring surgery, so it's essential to consult with a healthcare professional before making any decisions regarding treatment options. Factors like age, comorbidities, and individual risk tolerance should also be taken into consideration when deciding whether to pursue surgical intervention. Ultimately, the most effective treatment plan will depend on an evaluation of each patient's unique situation.

There are several reasons why surgical intervention might not be the best treatment option for heart disease. Firstly, some heart conditions can be managed effectively with medication alone, such as high blood pressure, coronary artery disease, and congenital heart defects. Secondly, heart surgery carries risks, including bleeding, infection, and complications related to anesthesia and other aspects of the procedure. Thirdly, some individuals may have underlying health issues that make them unsuitable candidates for surgery due to increased risk of adverse events or interactions with medications used during the procedure. Lastly, older adults and those with certain comorbidities may also be better suited for non-surgical treatments due to their lower ability to tolerate stress and recover from major surgery.

while surgery can be an effective treatment option for many types of heart disease, it's not the only option available. Patients must weigh the potential benefits and risks of surgical intervention against their individual circumstances and work closely with their healthcare providers to choose the best treatment path forward.

Chapter 11

IS THERE ANY RELATIONSHIP BETWEEN HEART DISEASE AND DIABETES

there is a strong link between heart disease and diabetes. Both conditions involve problems with circulation and metabolism. High glucose levels over time can damage the blood vessels and nerves, leading to cardiovascular disease and its complications. People with diabetes are at higher risk of developing heart disease, and vice versa. This is because both conditions increase the risk of inflammation, oxidative stress, and insulin resistance. Additionally, people with diabetes often have hypertension, dyslipidemia, obesity, sedentary lifestyle, smoking history, which are all known risk factors for heart disease. Therefore, managing both conditions together requires careful monitoring and coordination of medical care. Regular checkups, healthy diet, physical activity, and medication management are important for preventing and treating both heart disease and diabetes.

Relationship between heart disease and diabetes is complex, but one way to understand it is through the concept of endothelial dysfunction. Endothelium is the inner lining of blood vessels that regulates blood flow, helps maintain blood vessel integrity, and prevents clots. Over time, chronic hyperglycemia (high blood sugar) can lead to damage to endothelial cells, impairing their function and causing blood vessels to become stiff and narrowed. This leads to decreased blood flow, increased blood pressure, and an increased risk of plaque buildup, which can eventually lead to coronary artery disease and heart attack.

Another mechanism through which diabetes affects the heart is through inflammation and oxidative stress. Chronic elevated blood glucose levels can cause an accumulation of advanced glycation products (AGEs), which contribute to inflammation and oxidative stress in the body. These processes can lead to tissue damage and dysfunction, contributing to the development of heart disease.

Both diabetes and heart disease share common risk factors such as age, obesity, hypertension, dyslipidemia, and smoking history. All these factors contribute to systemic inflammation, oxidative stress, and insulin resistance, which further increases the risk of developing both conditions.

Therefore, it is crucial to manage both heart disease and diabetes simultaneously to reduce the risk of complications and improve overall health outcomes. This includes regular monitoring of blood glucose levels, blood pressure, cholesterol levels, and lipid profiles; maintaining a healthy diet, engaging in regular physical activity, quitting smoking, and taking prescribed medications as directed by healthcare professionals.

CHAPTER 12

CARDIAC CATHETERIZATION

Coronary angiography or cardiac catheterization is a diagnostic test used to evaluate the blood supply to the heart muscle and detect any blockages that may be present. It involves inserting a thin flexible tube called a catheter into a blood vessel in the wrist or groin and threading it up to the heart. Once inside the heart, contrast dye is injected through the catheter and X-ray images are taken to visualize the coronary arteries and identify any areas where they may be blocked. This information can then be used to guide treatment decisions, including whether surgery, balloon dilatation, or stents should be performed. Cardiac catheterization is typically done in a hospital setting and is considered a safe and effective procedure when used appropriately. However, like any medical procedure, it does carry some risks and potential side effects, such as bleeding, infection, allergic reactions, and heart attacks.

Coronary angiography or cardiac catheterization is a diagnostic test used to evaluate the blood supply to the heart muscle and detect any blockages that may be present. It involves inserting a thin flexible tube called a catheter into a blood vessel in the wrist or groin and threading it up to the heart. Once inside the heart, contrast dye is injected through the catheter and X-ray images are taken to visualize the coronary arteries and identify any areas where they may be blocked. This information can then be used to guide treatment decisions, including whether surgery, balloon dilatation, or stents should be performed. Cardiac catheterization is typically done in a hospital setting and is considered a safe and effective procedure when used appropriately. However, like any medical procedure, it does carry some risks and potential side effects, such as bleeding, infection, allergic reactions, and heart attacks.

Coronary angiography, commonly referred to as cardiac catheterization, has numerous benefits for patients suffering from heart disease. Here are some of the most significant advantages:

★Accuracy: Cardiac catheterization provides a precise and detailed image of the coronary arteries, allowing physicians to pinpoint any blockages, lesions, or other abnormalities that may be contributing to heart symptoms.

★Speed: The procedure typically takes less than two

hours, making it a fast and efficient way to diagnose and treat heart problems. This rapid turnaround time allows patients to receive prompt care and begin treatment sooner rather than later.

★ Safety: While there are always risks involved in any medical procedure, cardiac catheterization is considered relatively safe compared to other types of surgery or invasive treatments. In fact, many patients go home soon after the procedure without experiencing any major side effects.

★ Personalized Treatment: By identifying the specific areas of concern within the coronary arteries, cardiac catheterization enables physicians to tailor treatment plans to each individual patient. This personalized approach can help optimize results and reduce the likelihood of future complications.

★Improved Outcomes: Research consistently shows that patients who undergo cardiac catheterization experience better outcomes compared to those who do not receive the procedure. These improved outcomes include reduced rates of hospital readmissions, fewer recurrences of symptoms, and overall improvements in quality of life.

★ Cost-Effective: Although the initial cost of cardiac catheterization may seem daunting, studies have shown that the procedure can actually save money over the long term due to its ability to prevent more expensive surgeries and prolong life expectancy.

★Noninvasive Alternative: For some cases, cardiac catheterization serves as a noninvasive alternative to traditional surgical procedures. This lower-impact option can significantly reduce recovery times and alleviate concerns about scarring or tissue damage.

★Multidisciplinary Approach: Cardiac catheterization often requires collaboration among multiple healthcare professionals, such as cardiologists, radiologists, and interventionalists. This multidisciplinary teamwork ensures that patients receive comprehensive, coordinated care based on their unique needs and circumstances.

★Early Detection: By allowing physicians to diagnose heart issues at an early stage, cardiac catheterization facilitates timely intervention and prevention of further complications. This proactive approach can ultimately help delay or even avoid more severe health conditions down the line.

★Reduced Stress: Understanding your heart health and receiving appropriate treatment can greatly reduce stress levels and improve mental wellbeing. Knowledge empowers individuals to make informed decisions about their health and leads to greater peace of mind.

CHAPTER 13

OUTCOMES AND TYPES OF HEART DISEASE

★Cardiac Arrest

A cardiac arrest is a sudden cessation of the heart's ability to pump blood effectively due to an electrical or mechanical issue. It often occurs when there is a problem with the heart's rhythm (arrhythmia) or its structure (dysfunction). Cardiac arrest can be fatal if not treated promptly, as it leads to brain damage and death within minutes without oxygenation.

Symptoms of cardiac arrest may include sudden loss of consciousness, unresponsiveness, no breathing or gasping for air, chest pain, nausea, vomiting, and confusion. If you witness someone experiencing symptoms of cardiac arrest, call emergency medical services immediately and follow the instructions from trained personnel.

Cardiac arrest requires immediate resuscitation, usually through cardiopulmonary resuscitation (CPR), defibrillation, and possibly medications. During CPR, a trained rescuer will manually compress the heart using chest compression, providing artificial circulation while waiting for professional medical assistance. Defibrillation involves applying an electric shock to the heart to restore normal electrical activity and correct the arrhythmia.

The prognosis after a cardiac arrest depends on several factors, such as the duration of time between collapse and arrival at the hospital, the cause of the arrhythmia, and the presence of underlying conditions like diabetes, kidney disease, or respiratory problems. With rapid response, appropriate interventions, and ongoing care, some individuals may regain partial or full recovery. However, long-term survival rates are generally poor, with only about one in ten surviving beyond six months.

Prevention strategies for cardiac arrest include maintaining a healthy lifestyle, treating any pre-existing heart conditions, and addressing modifiable risk factors such as smoking, high blood pressure, obesity, and sedentary behavior. Regular exercise, maintaining a balanced diet, limiting alcohol intake, and avoiding certain drugs can also contribute to heart health and reduce the likelihood of cardiac arrest. Additionally, recognizing signs of an impending cardiac event and seeking medical attention promptly can increase chances of successful intervention and recovery.

Information About Cardiac Arrest

1. Types of Arrhythmias that Can Lead to Cardiac Arrest: There are various types of arrhythmias that can lead to cardiac arrest, including ventricular fibrillation (VF), ventricular tachycardia (VT), supraventricular tachycardia (SVT), atrial fibrillation

(AF), and bradycardia. VF and VT are the most common causes of cardiac arrest, accounting for approximately 80% of cases.

2. Causes of Cardiac Arrest: The causes of cardiac arrest can be categorized into congenital (present at birth), acquired (developed later in life), and iatrogenic (caused by medication or procedure) factors. Congenital disorders, such as hypertrophic cardiomyopathy (HCM), can weaken the heart muscle and make it susceptible to arrhythmias. Acquired factors, such as coronary artery disease, hyperlipidemia, hypertension, diabetes, and chronic lung diseases, can cause plaque buildup, narrowing of the arteries, and structural changes in the heart tissue. Iatrogenic factors include electrolyte imbalances, drug toxicities, and adverse reactions from surgical procedures or devices.

3. Risk Factors for Cardiac Arrest: Several risk factors have been identified for cardiac arrest, including age (older adults are at higher risk), gender (men are more likely than women), family history of sudden cardiac arrest or other heart conditions, smoking, alcohol consumption, lack of physical activity, poor diet, obesity, and sleep apnea. Chronic medical conditions, such as coronary artery disease, heart failure, valvular disorders, and abnormal rhythms, also increase the risk of cardiac arrest.

4. Treatment Options for Cardiac Arrest: Prompt

resuscitation and treatment are crucial for improving outcomes after cardiac arrest. The primary objective of initial treatment is to restore effective blood flow and oxygenation to vital organs. This is typically achieved through cardiopulmonary resuscitation (CPR) and defibrillation, as mentioned earlier. Additional interventions may include advanced cardiovascular life support (ACLS) techniques, medications (such as amiodarone, lidocaine, epinephrine, dobutamine, milrinone, and levosimendan), percutaneous coronary interventions (PCI), and surgical procedures (such as implantable loop recorders, pacemakers, defibrillators, and left ventricular assistive devices).

5. Outcomes After Cardiac Arrest: Survival rates after cardiac arres no urt depend on multiple factors, including the type and duration of the arrhythmia, the individual's overall health status, and the timely implementation of appropriate interventions. Rapid response, early detection, and efficient management of cardiac arrest significantly improve outcomes. While many patients recover with minimal neurological deficits, long-term complications can occur and vary depending on the severity and duration of the arrest, including cognitive impairment, mood disorders, anxiety, depression, posttraumatic stress disorder (PTSD), and functional limitations.

6. Prevention Strategies for Cardiac Arrest: To prevent cardiac arrest, maintain a healthy lifestyle by eating a

balanced diet, exercising regularly, managing chronic conditions, quitting smoking, and reducing alcohol consumption. Recognize warning signs of an impending cardiac event, such as chest discomfort, shortness of breath, dizziness, weakness, palpitations, or unexplained fatigue. Seek medical attention promptly if these symptoms arise. Finally, ensure proper training in cardiopulmonary resuscitation (CPR) and first aid skills among healthcare providers, family members, and community members to enhance the effectiveness of resuscitation efforts during a cardiac arrest.

Causes Of Cardiac Arrest

Cardiac arrest can be caused by several factors, which can be broadly classified into three categories: genetic or congenital, lifestyle and behavioral, and medical or physiological.

Genetic or congenital factors are inherited traits that predispose individuals to developing cardiac conditions leading to cardiac arrest. For example, some people inherit mutations that affect the heart muscles or electrical conduction system, increasing their risk of developing heart rhythm disturbances like ventricular tachycardia or ventricular fibrillation.

Lifestyle and behavioral factors contribute to cardiac arrest when they result in the development of underlying medical conditions. Examples of lifestyle and behavioral factors associated with increased risk of cardiac arrest include smoking, excessive alcohol intake, sedentary lifestyle, high salt intake, poor diet, and being overweight or obese.

Medical or physiological factors involve underlying health conditions that can progressively worsen over time and ultimately lead to cardiac arrest. These factors can be further subdivided into acute and chronic conditions. Acute conditions can develop rapidly and require immediate medical intervention, while chronic conditions can take years to manifest and can be managed through lifestyle modifications and ongoing medical care.

Some examples of medical or physiological factors causing cardiac arrest include coronary artery disease (CAD), hypertension (high blood pressure), diabetes mellitus, hyperthyroidism, hypothyroidism, sepsis (a severe infection), myocardial infarction (heart attack), pulmonary embolism (blood clot in the lungs), and electrolyte imbalances (abnormally low levels of minerals in the body fluids).

Overall, preventing cardiac arrest requires addressing

both genetic and lifestyle factors, as well as identifying and managing underlying medical conditions. Early recognition of warning signs and seeking medical help promptly can also save lives.

★Coronary artery disease

Coronary artery disease (CAD) is a type of heart disease that involves narrowing or blockage of the coronary arteries, which supply oxygenated blood to the heart muscle. This blockage reduces the amount of blood that flows to the heart muscle, limiting its ability to contract properly and increasing the risk of chest pain, heart attacks, strokes, and other cardiovascular problems. CAD is primarily caused by plaque buildup made up of cholesterol and other lipid particles in the walls of the coronary arteries. Over time, this buildup can form a hardened plaque layer, reducing blood flow to the heart and increasing the risk of cardiovascular disease.

Several risk factors associated with CAD, including

1. Age: The older population has a higher incidence of CAD compared to younger age groups.

2. Smoking: Smokers have a significantly higher risk of developing CAD than non-smokers due to the harmful effects of tobacco smoke on the heart and blood vessels.

3. Hyperlipidemia: High levels of bad cholesterols like low-density lipoprotein (LDL) and triglycerides increase the risk of plaque buildup and CAD.

4. Hypertension: Elevated blood pressure puts extra stress on the arteries, increasing the risk of plaque

formation and narrowing.

5. Diabetes: Both type 1 and type 2 diabetes increase the risk of CAD due to the damaging effect of high glucose levels on blood vessel function and inflammation.

6. Family history:

People with a family history of heart disease, particularly those who have had a relative diagnosed with CAD at a young age, have a higher risk of developing the condition themselves.

7. Obesity: Excess weight and belly fat can put additional strain on the heart and increase the risk of CAD.

The diagnosis of CAD typically involves non-invasive tests like electrocardiogram (ECG), echocardiography, and exercise stress testing. However, more invasive diagnostic procedures like angioplasty or coronary artery bypass surgery may be required in cases of advanced CAD or in situations where medication alone is insufficient to manage the condition.

Treatment options for CAD depend on the severity of the disease, individual patient factors, and overall health status. Medications like statins, aspirin, beta-blockers, and ACE inhibitors are commonly prescribed to manage CAD. Lifestyle interventions like smoking cessation, healthy eating, regular physical activity, and weight loss are also critical components of CAD management. In addition, surgical treatments like angioplasty, bypass surgery, and minimally invasive procedures like percutaneous coronary interventions (PCI) are used to restore normal blood flow to the heart in cases where medications and lifestyle changes are not sufficient.

Preventing CAD involves adopting healthy lifestyle habits and managing any underlying risk factors. Regular exercise, a balanced diet rich in fruits, vegetables, whole grains, lean protein, and healthy fats, maintaining a healthy weight, quitting smoking, and controlling conditions like high blood pressure and diabetes are all important steps in reducing the risk of CAD. Additionally, routine screenings and monitoring by healthcare providers can help detect CAD in its early stages, allowing for timely interventions and better outcomes.

★Heart failure

Heart failure is a type of heart disease characterized by the heart's inability to pump sufficient blood efficiently to meet the body's needs. In essence, the heart fails to maintain adequate circulation, leading to potential fluid retention and organ congestion, particularly in the lungs and legs. This condition usually develops gradually over time and can worsen without appropriate management.

Heart failure typically ensues due to damage or weakness to the heart muscle itself – often as a result of other underlying conditions like high blood pressure, diabetes, or coronary artery disease. The two primary types of heart failure include:

1. Systolic heart failure: This condition occurs when the heart cannot contract forcefully enough to eject sufficient blood out of its chambers during each beat, resulting in reduced output. This reduces the amount of blood available for the body, which can lead to symptoms such as shortness of breath and fatigue upon physical exertion.

2. Diastolic heart failure: Conversely, diastolic heart failure arises when the heart has trouble filling completely between beats. While it still contracts adequately, the stiffening of the ventricles hinders the intake of adequate blood into the heart chambers, ultimately compromising the overall efficiency of the circulatory system. Symptoms of diastolic heart failure are generally milder than those observed in systolic heart failure but might include fatigue, rapid breathing, and peripheral edema.

Regardless of whether someone experiences systolic or diastolic heart failure, the condition puts them at increased risk for hospitalization and premature death. Therefore, understanding the signs and symptoms of heart failure and taking proactive steps toward maintaining heart health is crucial. Consulting a healthcare professional for personalized advice is essential for individuals concerned about their heart health. Regular check-ups, adherence to prescribed treatments, healthy lifestyle choices, and ongoing monitoring can significantly improve outcomes for those living with heart failure.

Managing heart failure effectively involves several key aspects that aim to reduce symptoms, slow down disease progression, and enhance quality of life. Some common interventions for managing heart failure include:

1. Medications: A variety of medications may be prescribed to help manage heart failure, including:

  - Angiotensin-converting enzyme (ACE) inhibitors or angiotensin receptor blockers (ARBs): These drugs help dilate blood vessels, reducing strain on the heart and improving circulation.

  - Beta-blockers: By decreasing heart rate and

contractility, beta-blockers help the heart work more efficiently while also protecting against arrhythmias and sudden cardiac death.

- Diuretics: Prescribed to eliminate excess fluids from the body, thereby alleviating symptoms such as swelling in the legs and shortness of breath.

- Digoxin: A digitalis medication used to strengthen contractions and improve heart function.

- Aldosterone antagonists (mineralocorticoid receptor antagonists, MRAs): These drugs help regulate sodium and water balance within the body and prevent fluid accumulation.

2. Lifestyle modifications: Adopting certain lifestyle habits can contribute positively towards heart failure management, including:

- Diet: Consuming a low-sodium diet rich in fruits, vegetables, lean protein sources, whole grains, and heart-healthy fats helps support heart health.

- Physical activity: Engaging in regular aerobic activities like walking or cycling can boost cardiovascular fitness, improve energy levels, and aid in weight control.

- Weight management: Keeping a healthy weight can decrease stress on the heart and ease the burden on the heart muscle.

- Rest and relaxation techniques: Techniques such as deep breathing exercises, meditation, and progressive muscle relaxation can promote emotional calmness and better cardiovascular function.

- Limiting alcohol consumption: Alcohol should be consumed moderately (if at all), as excessive drinking can negatively impact heart function.

3. Monitoring symptoms and tracking progress: Close collaboration with healthcare professionals is vital for effective heart failure management. Self-monitoring techniques like daily weighing, recording fluid intake and output, and assessing symptom severity can enable timely adjustments to treatment plans.

4. Regular follow-up appointments: Regular check-ups allow medical personnel to evaluate the effectiveness of current therapies and make necessary alterations to optimize treatment plans.

5. Education and support groups: Acquiring knowledge about heart failure and connecting with others dealing with similar challenges can provide valuable insights, emotional encouragement, and practical tips for coping with the condition. Many resources and organizations offer educational materials and

networking opportunities tailored specifically to people living with heart failure.

★Pericardial Disease

Pericardial diseases refer to conditions affecting the pericardium – the thin sac surrounding the heart. The pericardium plays a crucial role in protecting the heart and maintaining its proper functioning through lubrication and regulation of pressure. Several pericardial disorders exist, each presenting unique characteristics and management approaches. Here's an overview of some common pericardial diseases:

1. Pericarditis: Inflammation of the pericardium, most commonly caused by viral infection but sometimes due to bacterial, fungal, tuberculosis, or other underlying conditions. Symptoms include chest pain (sharp, stabbing or dull, worsened by lying flat or taking deep breaths), fever, shortness of breath, and palpitations. Treatment often involves nonsteroidal anti-inflammatory drugs (NSAIDs), colchicine, corticosteroids, antibiotics if an infectious cause is suspected, and supportive care.

2. Pericardial effusion: Accumulation of fluid within the pericardial space, which can put pressure on the heart leading to various symptoms like chest pain, shortness of breath, and pulsus paradoxus. Causes range from idiopathic causes to malignancies,

connective tissue diseases, kidney failure, or uremia. Depending upon the size and nature of the effusion, treatments include diuretics, pericentesis, surgery, or sclerosant instillation into the pericardial sac.

3. Constrictive pericarditis: Scarring and thickening of the pericardium results in loss of compliance, causing impaired filling of the ventricles during diastole. This chronic condition usually follows acute pericarditis and presents with symptoms like fatigue, weight loss, dyspnea, peripheral edema, abdominal distension, and hepatosplenomegaly. Management includes corticosteroids, non-steroidal anti-inflammatory agents, diuretics, and pericardiectomy (surgical removal of the restrictive layers).

Strategies For Managing Pericardial Disease

Pericardial diseases require careful evaluation and appropriate intervention for effective management. The choice of therapy depends largely on the specific type and severity of the disease. Here's a brief overview of possible interventions for three common types of pericardial diseases:

1. Pericarditis:

- Nonsteroidal Anti-Inflammatory Drugs (NSAIDs) or Colchicine: These medications help reduce inflammation and alleviate chest pain.

- Corticosteroids: For severe cases that do not respond adequately to NSAIDs or colchicine, corticosteroids may be prescribed to decrease inflammation and speed up recovery.

- Antibiotics: If there is suspicion of a bacterial etiology, antibiotics will be administered accordingly.

- Supportive Care: Fluid and electrolyte replacement, as well as oxygen supplementation, might be necessary in certain cases to manage symptoms and maintain cardiac function.

2. Pericardial Effusion:

- Diuretics: To manage excess fluid accumulation, diuretics may be used to encourage urination and help alleviate symptoms such as shortness of breath and congestion.

- Pericentesis: A procedure where a small amount of fluid is removed from the pericardial sac using a needle, allowing relief from compression on the heart and improved breathing. Repeated procedures may be needed in recurrent cases.

- Surgery: Surgical options like pericardectomy or window creation can be considered for large effusions resistant to medical therapy or those associated with complications such as tamponade.

- Sclerosants: Instillation of sclerosants directly into the pericardial sac can promote fibrosis and scar formation, helping seal off the leaking area and prevent further effusion.

3. Constrictive Pericarditis:

- Corticosteroids: High doses of oral corticosteroids can help improve symptoms in constrictive pericarditis, though long term use carries risks like side effects and potential dependency.

- Non-Steroidal Anti-Inflammatory Agents: Low dose aspirin or ibuprofen may be given to minimize inflammation and discomfort.

- Diuretics: These medicines assist in removing excess fluid build-up around the lungs and body, thus reducing symptoms like shortness of breath and swelling.

- Pericardiectomy: When all else fails, surgically removing the affected portions of the pericardium allows normal heart movement and improves overall cardiac functionality.

Please note this information serves only as a general guide, and individualized management plans should be determined through consultation with healthcare professionals. Additionally, early recognition and prompt treatment significantly enhance outcomes for individuals diagnosed with these pericardial diseases.

★valvular heart disease

Valvular heart disease refers to conditions that affect the heart valves, preventing them from functioning properly. Proper valve function is crucial for maintaining an adequate blood flow between the chambers of the heart and ensuring efficient circulation throughout the body. Several factors contribute to valvular heart disease, including age, genetics, infection, and connective tissue disorders. There are various types of valvular heart diseases, each requiring unique approaches for management.

1. Mitral Stenosis: This condition involves narrowing or stiffening of the mitral valve, which obstructs blood flow from the left atrium into the left ventricle. Symptoms include shortness of breath, fatigue, irregular heartbeat, and edema in the legs and feet due to poor circulation. Treatment includes balloon valvuloplasty, surgical repair or replacement of the damaged valve, and anticoagulation therapy for those at risk of developing clots.

2. Aortic Stenosis: Characterized by narrowing or calcification of the aortic valve, aortic stenosis impedes blood flow leaving the left ventricle. Symptoms include chest pain, shortness of breath, fainting episodes, and heart palpitations. Treatments include balloon valvuloplasty, transcatheter aortic valve implantation (TAVI), or surgical replacement of the aortic valve.

3. Mitral Regurgitation: In this condition, the mitral valve does not close properly, causing regurgitation or leakage of blood from the left ventricle back into the left atrium during systole. Causes range from degenerative changes to damage resulting from rheumatic fever or myocardial infarction. Management strategies include medications to control symptoms like hypertension and heart failure; surgery for symptomatic patients, and occasionally, repair via minimally invasive procedures.

4. Tricuspid Stenosis or Regurgitation: Both tricuspid stenosis and regurgitation involve malfunctioning of the right heart's tricuspid valve. Symptoms depend on the extent of obstruction or leakage but often include fatigue, shortness of breath, swollen abdomen, and lower extremity edema. Conservative treatments

include salt restriction, diuretics, and digitalis glycosides. Severe cases necessitate surgical repair or replacement of the tricuspid valve.

Regardless of the specific type of valvular heart disease, timely diagnosis and appropriate intervention are essential for optimizing patient outcomes. It's important to consult healthcare professionals for accurate assessment and personalized care plans.

Strategies for preventing Valvular heart disease

While there are no foolproof methods to prevent valvular heart disease entirely, certain measures can help reduce the risks associated with its development and progression. Here are some recommendations for prevention and management:

1. Regular check-ups and screenings: Regular medical evaluations, especially for individuals with known risk factors such as advanced age, family history, hypertension, diabetes, or other chronic health conditions, can help identify early signs of valvular heart disease.

2. Healthy lifestyle habits: Adopting healthy lifestyle choices, such as regular physical activity, balanced nutrition, stress reduction techniques, and avoidance of tobacco use and excessive alcohol consumption, may decrease your chances of developing valvular heart disease or worsening existing conditions.

3. Controlling underlying conditions: Effectively managing conditions like high blood pressure, diabetes, and hyperlipidemia through medication, diet, and exercise can help slow down the progression of valvular heart disease.

4. Preventive antibiotics prior to dental procedures: For people with certain types of valvular heart disease – particularly those who have had previous endocarditis or artificial heart valves – taking antibiotics before undergoing dental procedures can help minimize the risk of infective endocarditis. Consult your doctor about whether you need preventive antibiotics.

5. Close monitoring and follow-up care: If diagnosed with valvular heart disease, it's crucial to adhere strictly to prescribed treatment plans and attend routine appointments with your healthcare team to

monitor the disease's progression and adjust therapies accordingly.

6.Consider surgical interventions when necessary: When noninvasive treatments prove insufficient, your healthcare provider might recommend surgical options like valve repairs or replacements to improve cardiac functionality and overall quality of life. These surgeries offer significant benefits for many patients living with severe valvular heart disease.

★Cardiomyopathy

Cardiomyopathy is a group of diseases that affect the structure and function of the heart muscle. The condition weakens the ability of the heart to pump efficiently, making it harder for the organ to supply enough oxygenated blood throughout the body. There are several types of cardiomyopathy, including:

1. Dilated cardiomyopathy - Characterized by an enlarged left ventricle (the main pumping chamber of the heart) that becomes less effective at pushing blood out effectively.

2. Hypertrophic cardiomyopathy - Involving abnormal thickening of the heart muscle, which impairs the

heart's ability to fill properly between beats.

3. Restrictive cardiomyopathy - Resulting from a stiffened, inflexible heart wall, making it difficult for the heart to fill adequately during diastole (relaxation phase).

4. Idiopathic restrictive cardiomyopathy - A rare type caused by unknown reasons, characterized by decreased compliance and reduced filling capacity due to various causes not related to the heart muscle itself.

5. Ischemic cardiomyopathy - Damage to the heart muscle caused by a lack of blood flow and oxygen leading to scarring and fibrosis, often following a myocardial infarction (heart attack).

Common symptoms of cardiomyopathy include shortness of breath, fatigue, swelling in the legs, ankles, and feet, irregular heartbeat, and fluid retention in the lungs or abdomen. Treatment options range from medications and lifestyle modifications to surgery and transplantation depending on the severity and cause of the condition. It is essential to consult a healthcare professional if experiencing any concerning symptoms to receive appropriate diagnosis and guidance.

Cardiomyopathy is a group of diseases that affect the structure and function of the heart muscle. The condition weakens the ability of the heart to pump efficiently, making it harder for the organ to supply enough oxygenated blood throughout the body. There are several types of cardiomyopathy, including:

1. Dilated cardiomyopathy - Characterized by an enlarged left ventricle (the main pumping chamber of the heart) that becomes less effective at pushing blood out effectively.

2. Hypertrophic cardiomyopathy - Involving abnormal thickening of the heart muscle, which impairs the heart's ability to fill properly between beats.

3. Restrictive cardiomyopathy - Resulting from a stiffened, inflexible heart wall, making it difficult for the heart to fill adequately during diastole (relaxation phase).

4. Idiopathic restrictive cardiomyopathy - A rare type caused by unknown reasons, characterized by decreased compliance and reduced filling capacity due to various causes not related to the heart muscle itself.

5. Ischemic cardiomyopathy - Damage to the heart muscle caused by a lack of blood flow and oxygen leading to scarring and fibrosis, often following a

myocardial infarction (heart attack).

Common symptoms of cardiomyopathy include shortness of breath, fatigue, swelling in the legs, ankles, and feet, irregular heartbeat, and fluid retention in the lungs or abdomen. Treatment options range from medications and lifestyle modifications to surgery and transplantation depending on the severity and cause of the condition. It is essential to consult a healthcare professional if experiencing any concerning symptoms to receive appropriate diagnosis and guidance.

Strategies For Preventing Cardiomyopathy

Although there are no definitive ways to completely prevent cardiomyopathy since many cases are caused by genetic or inherited factors or preexisting conditions, certain steps can help lower your risk:

1. Heart-healthy lifestyle: Eating a nutritious diet rich in fruits, vegetables, whole grains, lean proteins, and omega-3 fatty acids while avoiding saturated fats and trans fats; maintaining a healthy weight; engaging in regular physical activity; reducing stress levels; and quitting smoking are all important for promoting heart health.

2. Management of pre-existing conditions: Properly controlling chronic conditions such as high blood

pressure, diabetes, and obesity can significantly reduce the risk of developing cardiomyopathy. Ensure timely detection and prompt treatment of these conditions through regular check-ups and following the recommended therapy plan.

3. Avoiding harmful substances: Limiting alcohol intake and avoiding illicit drugs like cocaine and amphetamines, which can lead to damage of the heart muscle and increase the likelihood of developing cardiomyopathy.

4. Screening and early intervention: People with a family history of cardiomyopathy should consider getting regular screening tests to detect potential issues earlier and seek medical advice for early intervention. This could involve close monitoring of heart function through echocardiograms and electrocardiograms.

5. Medications: Some medications, such as beta blockers and angiotensin-converting enzyme inhibitors, have been shown to protect against cardiomyopathy by improving blood flow and reducing strain on the heart. Your healthcare provider can assess if these medications are suitable for your

specific situation.

6. Monitoring symptoms closely: Pay attention to warning signs such as chest pain, palpitations, and shortness of breath. Report any new or worsening symptoms to your healthcare professional immediately, as early recognition and treatment can make a difference in outcomes for individuals with cardiomyopathy.

7. Regular exercise: Engaging in moderate intensity aerobic activities like brisk walking, cycling, swimming, or gardening for at least 150 minutes per week has proven beneficial for heart health. Always consult your physician before starting a new exercise regimen, especially if you already have cardiovascular concerns.

★Arrhythmia

Arrhythmia refers to an irregular heart rhythm or an abnormal electrical conduction system within the heart. The normal sequence of electrical impulses that coordinate heart contractions may become disrupted, leading to various types of arrhythmias such as atrial fibrillation, atrial flutter, ventricular tachycardia, and ventricular fibrillation. These conditions can range from harmless, causing only minor symptoms, to life-threatening.

Risk factors for arrhythmias include:

1. Pre-existing heart conditions (such as coronary artery disease, hypertension, valvular heart diseases)

2. Age

3. Genetics

4. Electrolyte imbalances (potassium, sodium, calcium, magnesium)

5. Use of certain medications (beta blockers, diuretics, thyroid hormones, etc.)

6. Substance abuse (alcohol, caffeine, tobacco)

7. Obstructive sleep apnea

8. Stress and emotional disorders

9. Hormonal changes (during pregnancy, menopause, etc.)

10. Infections (rheumatic fever, bacterial endocarditis, Lyme disease)

Symptoms associated with arrhythmias may include:

1. Palpitations (feeling that the heart is pounding, racing, skipping beats, or flip-flopping)

2. Shortness of breath

3. Dizziness or lightheadedness

4. Chest pain

5. Weakness

6. Rapid breathing or pulse

7. Fatigue

8. Fainting or near-fainting episodes

9. Swelling in legs, feet, or stomach due to fluid retention

10. Confusion or memory problems

If experiencing any arrhythmia symptoms, it's essential to consult a doctor for proper diagnosis and treatment recommendations. Treatment options depend on the type and severity of the arrhythmia and may consist of medications, procedures (catheter ablation), surgery, or implantable devices like pacemakers or automatic implantable cardioverter-defibrillators (AICD). Adherence to heart-healthy lifestyle practices, including regular exercise, eating balanced meals, managing stress, and avoiding harmful substances, also plays a crucial role in minimizing the risk of developing arrhythmias.

Arrhythmias are common heart conditions affecting millions of people worldwide. They occur when there is an issue with the electrical signals in the heart, which disrupt the usual sequence of contractions necessary for effective blood circulation. Arrhythmias can affect both the upper chambers (atria) and lower chambers (ventricles) of the heart.

Atrial arrhythmias involve the atria, while ventricular arrhythmias primarily impact the ventricles. Atrial fibrillation (AFib) is one of the most prevalent types of atrial arrhythmias. During AFib, the atria quiver rather than contract effectively, allowing small amounts of blood to pool inside these chambers. This condition increases the risk of clots forming, which can potentially lead to stroke if they travel to the brain. Symptoms of atrial arrhythmias include palpitations, shortness of breath, dizziness, weakness, fatigue, chest pain, rapid breathing, and confusion.

Ventricular arrhythmias originate from the ventricles and can cause serious consequences. One such example is ventricular fibrillation (VFib), where the heart stops pumping efficiently due to chaotic electrical activity. VFib often results in loss of consciousness and sudden cardiac arrest. Other ventricular arrhythmias, such as premature ventricular contractions (PVCs), might not present significant symptoms but could increase the risk of more dangerous arrhythmias.

Treatment approaches for arrhythmias vary depending on their underlying causes, severity, and impact on daily living. For mild cases, lifestyle modifications – such as maintaining a healthy weight, exercising regularly, reducing stress, and following a balanced diet – may help manage or even prevent arrhythmias. Medications like beta-blockers, antiarrhythmic drugs, and anticoagulants play crucial roles in treating specific arrhythmias, preventing complications, and restoring regular heart rhythms.

Invasive interventions, such as catheter ablation and surgery, are used for severe or drug-resistant arrhythmias. Catheter ablation involves using heat, cold, or other energy sources to destroy tiny areas of heart tissue responsible for triggering erratic heartbeats. Surgical treatments include maze procedure, Mini-Maze, and Cox maze surgery. These methods create scarring inside the heart to disrupt the pathways causing arrhythmias.

Implantable devices like pacemakers and AICDs offer lifesaving solutions for individuals who experience recurrent arrhythmias or have a higher risk of sudden death due to cardiac conditions. Pacemakers generate electrical impulses to maintain correct heart rhythms when natural beats fail to occur, whereas AICDs deliver electric shocks to restore normal heart function during life-threatening ventricular arrhythmias.

It's important to remember that everyone's situation is unique. If you suspect having an arrhythmia, seeking medical advice promptly is essential. Regular checkups, especially for those with pre-existing heart conditions, age, or family history, are crucial for early detection and effective management of potential arrhythmias.

CHAPTER 14

Cardiac Electrophysiology And Pacing Therapies

Cardiac electrophysiology is a subspecialty of cardiology focused on diagnosing and managing heart rhythm disorders, commonly known as arrhythmias. It deals with the study of electrical properties and conduction systems within the heart, aiming to identify the underlying mechanisms behind various heart rhythm disturbances.

The primary goal of cardiac electrophysiology is to understand the complex interactions between electrical signals and ion channels in the heart. Electrophysiological studies employ invasive techniques like catheter ablation and non-invasive tests, such as ambulatory ECG monitoring and echocardiography, to evaluate patients' hearts and assess their response to treatment.

One critical area of research and clinical application within cardiac electrophysiology is pacing therapies. Pacing therapy refers to interventions aimed at maintaining appropriate heart rates and restoring normal heart rhythms through artificial means. The two main pacing modalities are:

1. External pacing: In this method, an external device delivers electrical impulses directly to the heart via large electrodes placed on the patient's chest. External pacemakers are typically employed as temporary measures in emergencies or during diagnostic procedures to maintain adequate cardiac

output.

2. Implantable pacing systems: Modern implantable pacing systems consist of a battery-powered pulse generator connected to electrode leads positioned within the heart chambers. Once surgically implanted under local anesthesia, these devices regulate the heart's beating by generating electrical pulses when the native heart rhythm falls below a set threshold. There are three primary types of implantable pacemakers:

- Single chamber pacemaker: This system only senses and stimulates a single chamber (usually the right ventricle). It is suitable for patients requiring basic pacing needs.

- Dual chamber pacemaker: With two electrode leads, dual chamber pacemakers monitor and pace both the right atrium and right ventricle, ensuring synchronization between the two chambers for improved efficiency and better mimicking of physiologic heart contractions.

- Biventricular pacemaker: In addition to controlling both atria and ventricles separately, biventricular pacemakers provide synchronized stimulation to optimize cardiac contraction, particularly beneficial for patients diagnosed with heart failure or certain arrhythmias.

Advanced pacing technologies include adaptive rate pacing algorithms designed to adjust pacing parameters according to individual requirements and multisite pacing strategies that target multiple sites within the heart chambers for enhanced coordination and improved outcomes. Additionally, ongoing advancements in wireless communication technology enable remote programming and monitoring capabilities for greater flexibility and convenience.

Cardiac resynchronization therapy (CRT) represents another innovative pacing intervention tailored specifically for patients suffering from advanced heart failure. By delivering precisely timed electrical impulses to both left and right ventricles simultaneously, CRT aims to restore proper timing and coordination among heart muscle groups, leading to improvements in cardiac performance, exercise capacity, and overall quality of life.

As technology advances, pacing therapies continue to evolve, offering new opportunities for personalized care and optimal outcomes for patients dealing with various heart rhythm disorders. Continuous research and development will undoubtedly contribute significantly to refining our understanding of cardiac electrophysiology and expanding the therapeutic arsenal available to clinicians addressing these complex conditions.

Let me expand on some aspects of cardiac electrophysiology and pacing therapies, focusing on recent developments and future directions.

1. Innovations in pacing technologies: Researchers and engineers continue pushing the boundaries of pacing therapy by exploring novel technologies that enhance the effectiveness, safety, and user experience of existing devices. Some exciting innovations include:

  * Leadless pacemakers: These tiny, self-contained pacemakers eliminate the need for thoracotomy surgery and reduce complications associated with traditional lead-based systems. They are implanted using minimally invasive methods, such as transcatheter delivery through the vena cava.

  * Magnetic resonance imaging (MRI)-compatible pacemakers: As many patients require regular MRIs, developing pacemakers capable of functioning inside the strong magnetic field without interference has become crucial. Recent advancements have made MRI-safe pacemakers increasingly common.

- Closed-loop pacing: A closed-loop pacing system uses real-time sensing and analysis of intracardiac pressure changes and other hemodynamic variables to automatically adjust pacing output, enabling more efficient energy utilization and potentially improving patient outcomes.

- Long-term rechargeable batteries: Current pacemaker batteries generally last around 8-10 years before replacement; however, efforts are being made to develop long-lasting, rechargeable alternatives. Such batteries could offer significant advantages, including reduced procedure frequency, lower costs, and environmental sustainability.

2. Personalized medicine approaches: Precision medicine holds great promise for transforming cardiac electrophysiology and pacing therapies. By leveraging genomic information, biomarkers, and lifestyle factors, healthcare providers can tailor treatments to each patient's unique condition, ensuring maximum benefit and minimum risk. For example, pharmacogenomics can help determine which medications would be most effective for specific patients based on their genetic makeup, while wearable health monitors and telehealth tools can facilitate remote tracking of vital signs and symptoms, allowing for earlier detection and prompt intervention.

3. Artificial intelligence and machine learning applications: Machine learning algorithms and artificial intelligence (AI) can analyze vast amounts of data generated by pacemakers, electronic health records, and other sources to uncover hidden patterns, predict potential complications, and inform personalized treatment plans. Applications range from automated event recognition, risk stratification, and prognosis assessment to intelligent decision support systems and autonomous treatment recommendations, ultimately empowering doctors to make more informed choices and improve patient experiences.

4. Advancements in ablation techniques: Catheter ablation remains a cornerstone of arrhythmia management, and technological progress continues in this realm as well. Enhancement of mapping systems, development of contact force sensors, and integration of AI algorithms into ablation platforms allow for more precise and efficient elimination of abnormal electrical pathways, reducing procedural risks and recurrence rates. Furthermore, combining ablation with other interventional modalities, such as left atrial appendage closure or valvular repair, can broaden the scope of what can be achieved in a single session, simplifying follow-up treatments and

streamlining workflows.

Cardiac electrophysiology and pacing therapies represent dynamic fields that are constantly advancing through innovation, collaboration, and scientific discovery. From cutting-edge technologies and personalized approaches to improved diagnostics and targeted interventions, the future looks bright for those seeking solutions to complex heart rhythm disorders. Ultimately, the goal is to deliver safer, more effective, and convenient treatments that cater to the diverse needs of individuals living with cardiovascular conditions.

CHAPTER 15

Advance Heart Monitoring Techniques

Advance heart monitoring techniques refer to the latest technologies and methods used for continuous or intermittent assessment of cardiac function and rhythm. These techniques go beyond traditional electrocardiograms (ECG) and Holter monitors, providing more detailed and comprehensive information about the heart's condition. Some advanced heart monitoring techniques include:

1. Ambulatory Blood Pressure Monitoring (ABPM): This noninvasive technique involves wearing a device that measures blood pressure at regular intervals throughout the day. It provides a better understanding of blood pressure changes over an extended period than office readings. ABPM is particularly useful for diagnosing hypertension, sleep apnea, and white coat syndrome.

2. Echocardiography: An echocardiogram uses sound waves to create images of the heart chambers and their structures. The test evaluates the size and shape of various parts of the heart and assesses its pumping capacity. Stress echocardiography adds

exercise stressors like treadmill or bicycle ergometry to determine how the heart functions during physical activity.

3. Cardiac Magnetic Resonance Imaging (MRI): Cardiac MRIs use strong magnetic fields and radio waves to generate detailed pictures of the heart and its structures. They allow doctors to evaluate the heart's function, identify abnormalities, such as tumors or scarring, and measure the extent of damage caused by conditions like coronary artery disease.

4. Electrophysiology studies: In this invasive procedure, thin tubes called catheters are inserted into a vein in your arm or groin area, guided through the blood vessels to your heart. Doctors then record electrical signals from inside your heart while applying stimuli to assess the heart's conduction system. This helps diagnose arrhythmias and plan treatment options like catheter ablation.

5. Telemonitoring: Remote heart monitoring allows patients with chronic heart diseases to monitor their vital signs, including heart rate and blood pressure, at home using wireless devices. The data is transmitted electronically to healthcare providers who analyze it remotely and provide timely advice or adjust

medication accordingly.

6. Wearable Heart Rate Variability Monitors: These portable devices continuously track heart rate variability - the natural fluctuation in heartbeats' interval between beats. A decrease in heart rate variability may indicate increased sympathetic nervous system activity and predict worsening health status in individuals with heart failure or other conditions.

7. Continuous Glucose Monitoring Systems: While primarily designed for diabetes management, these systems can also help detect sudden drops in glucose levels that might trigger life-threatening arrhythmias in people with underlying heart problems.

CHAPTER 16

TRANSCATHETER AORTIC VALVE REPLACEMENT (TAVR)

Transcatheter Aortic Valve Replacement (TAVR) is a minimally invasive procedure that has significantly transformed the landscape of treating severe aortic stenosis - a condition characterized by narrowing of the aortic valve opening. TAVR represents an alternative to traditional open-heart surgery (aortic valve replacement) for individuals who may not be suitable candidates due to age, comorbidities, or risk factors.

In this procedure, a specialist threadedly inserts a collapsed balloon-expandable or self-expanding bioprosthetic heart valve through a small incision in the leg or chest, typically via the femoral artery. Once positioned correctly in the diseased valve, the new valve expands, replacing the native valve and restoring proper blood flow from the left ventricle to the aorta. The delivery system is then removed, leaving only the newly implanted valve behind.

The advantages of TAVR include reduced surgical trauma compared to open-heart surgery, shorter hospital stays, faster recovery times, lower mortality rates, and decreased morbidity. Additionally, TAVR can provide substantial quality-of-life improvements as it alleviates symptoms such as shortness of breath and chest pain commonly associated with aortic stenosis.

However, there are certain considerations and risks associated with TAVR, including the possibility of complications such as bleeding at the access site, stroke, acute kidney injury, and paravalvular leakage. It is important to weigh these risks against the benefits of improved hemodynamics and symptom relief provided by the procedure.

Despite its advantages, TAVR remains a complex intervention requiring expertise in image guidance, vessel access, valve sizing, and positioning. Ongoing research aims to expand the indications for TAVR while continuously refining procedural techniques to optimize safety and efficacy.

Transcatheter aortic valve replacement represents a major breakthrough in the field of structural heart interventions, providing an increasingly viable option for high-risk patients suffering from severe aortic stenosis. With continued advances and improvements in technology, TAVR is poised to revolutionize the way we approach valve replacement procedures, offering hope and better outcomes to those living with debilitating aortic valve diseases.

Transcatheter Aortic Valve Replacement (TAVR) has emerged as a game-changer in the treatment of severe aortic stenosis, especially for those patients who are considered high risk for conventional open-heart surgery due to advanced age, multiple comorbidities, or other health concerns. This innovative procedure offers several advantages over traditional valve replacement surgeries:

★Minimally Invasive: One of the most significant benefits of TAVR lies in its minimally invasive nature. Instead of making a large incision in the chest, specialists perform the procedure using a catheter inserted either through a small incision in the groin or the upper thigh. This reduces overall tissue damage and results in quicker healing time.

★Reduced Hospital Stays: Since TAVR is less invasive than open-heart surgery, patients usually spend fewer days in the hospital following the procedure. Shorter hospitalization periods contribute to both cost savings and increased patient comfort.

★ Faster Recovery Time: TAVR boasts rapid recovery times compared to traditional valve replacement surgeries. Patients often experience minimal discomfort and regain mobility much sooner after undergoing the procedure.

★Lower Mortality Rates: TAVR has been shown to have lower mortality rates when compared to surgery in select patient populations, particularly older adults and those with complex medical conditions.

★Improved Quality of Life: By restoring proper blood flow from the left ventricle to the aorta, TAVR provides substantial quality-of-life improvements for many patients. Symptoms such as chest pain, shortness of breath, fatigue, and swelling in the legs and ankles caused by aortic stenosis are often substantially relieved after successful TAVR procedures.

★Continuous Advancements: As research progresses, TAVR continues to evolve. New innovations focus on expanding indications for the procedure and improving its safety and efficiency. For example, the development of self-expanding valves and advancements in imaging technologies have made it possible to treat even more complex cases. Furthermore, ongoing clinical trials aim to determine the long-term durability and effectiveness of various TAVR devices.

★ Cost Effectiveness: While the initial investment required for TAVR technology might seem high, the procedure's potential for reducing hospitalizations, rehospitalizations, and lengthy recoveries makes it cost effective in the long run. Over time, TAVR could save healthcare systems significant resources by streamlining the treatment process and enabling earlier return to normal activities for patients.

★Global Impact: TAVR holds immense promise for addressing the global burden of valve disease. According to the World Health Organization, approximately 2% of people aged 70 years and above suffer from aortic stenosis, but only a fraction receive adequate care due to limited resources and accessibility issues. TAVR presents an opportunity to bring life-changing treatments to millions of patients worldwide.

★Expanding Applications: Initially designed primarily for elderly patients and those deemed too high risk for surgery, TAVR is now being studied for use in younger patients with less severe aortic stenosis. These developments may broaden the application spectrum and make TAVR accessible to a larger population in need of valve replacement therapy.

★Future Perspectives: The future looks promising for TAVR. Innovative approaches like supra-annular, sub-annular, and annuloplasty ring designs continue to emerge, potentially enhancing the device's performance and longevity. Moreover, combination therapies involving TAVR alongside additional interventional procedures like coronary revascularization or atrial fibrillation ablation hold great promise for improving patient outcomes. Ultimately, TAVR stands to transform cardiovascular medicine, empowering physicians to address a wide range of valve disorders in a safer, more efficient manner.

Transcatheter Aortic Valve Replacement (TAVR) has been a game-changer in the treatment of aortic valve disease, particularly in older adults or those with significant comorbidities who are unable or unwilling to undergo open-heart surgery. Traditional surgical aortic valve replacement involves opening the chest and stopping the heart to replace the damaged valve. This process carries inherent risks, including prolonged hospital stays, lengthy recoveries, and potential complications.

TAVR offers several advantages over surgical valve replacement:

1. Minimally Invasive: Instead of making a large incision, physicians use a catheter – a thin tube – to deliver the new valve to the affected area. This technique results in less tissue damage and reduces postoperative pain.

2. Shorter Hospital Stays: Patients typically spend fewer days in the hospital after undergoing TAVR than they would following surgical valve replacement. This not only helps reduce healthcare costs but also enables quicker return home and resumption of daily activities.

3. Quicker Recovery Times: With minimal invasiveness comes a swifter recovery period. TAVR patients often experience less discomfort and regain

their energy levels sooner than those recovering from open-heart surgery.

4. Lower Mortality Rates: Clinical studies have shown that TAVR is associated with lower mortality rates when compared to surgical valve replacement in specific patient populations. This makes it an attractive choice for individuals whose health conditions make them higher-risk candidates for surgery.

5. Quality-of-Life Improvements: Severe aortic stenosis can cause symptoms like shortness of breath, fatigue, chest pain, and difficulty performing routine tasks. TAVR addresses these concerns by improving hemodynamic function and relieving the symptoms caused by a failing aortic valve, ultimately enhancing overall quality of life.

While TAVR holds many benefits, it does carry some risks. Some common complications include:

1. Access Site Bleeding: As the procedure requires insertion through an artery in the leg or chest, there's a chance for bleeding at the puncture site. This could potentially lead to further complications if the bleed continues unchecked.

2. Stroke: Though rare, the risk of having a stroke increases slightly after TAVR due to the presence of a foreign object within the body. This risk factor should be considered during decision-making about whether

TAVR is the best course of action.

3. Acute Kidney Injury: Occasionally, TAVR can result in temporary or permanent loss of kidney function. This occurs because of the increased pressure exerted on the kidneys during the procedure or the use of contrast dye, which can harm kidney cells.

4. Paravalvular Leakage: In some cases, tiny leaks can form around the edges of the prosthetic valve. These leaks might require additional intervention to prevent serious consequences, such as endocarditis or further deterioration of heart function.

It's essential to remember that each individual case is unique; therefore, the benefits and risks vary depending on various factors such as age, medical history, and overall health status. Close collaboration between cardiologists, interventionalists, radiologists, and other healthcare professionals plays a crucial role in ensuring optimal outcomes for every TAVR patient.

Continuous advancements in technology continue to push the boundaries of what's possible in Transcatheter Aortic Valve Replacement. Researchers and clinicians work tirelessly to improve upon existing techniques, expand indication criteria, and develop newer, safer devices designed specifically for TAVR procedures. By addressing both current challenges and future needs, the goal is to ensure that this innovative procedure remains a valuable tool in the ongoing fight against aortic valve disease and improves the lives of countless individuals worldwide.

CHAPTER 17

EFFECTIVE ALTERNATIVE AND COMPLEMENTARY THERAPIES FOR HEART HEALTH

I'm glad you're interested in heart health! There are several alternative and complementary therapies that have been suggested to support a healthy cardiovascular system. Here are some of them:

Let me expand on some of these alternative and complementary therapies for heart health and provide additional insights.

★Meditative practices such as mindfulness meditation, yoga, and Transcendental Meditation (TM) are powerful tools to manage stress, which is a major risk factor for heart diseases. Regular practice can lead to reduced inflammation, improved immune response, lower blood pressure, and enhanced cardiac autonomic tone. These practices also contribute positively to overall mental and emotional wellbeing.

★Aromatherapy with essential oils is a simple yet effective way to incorporate relaxation and self-care into daily routines. Essential oils can be diffused in rooms, applied topically diluted with carrier oils, or added to bathwater. When selecting essential oils, make sure to purchase certified pure therapeutic-grade oils, as inferior quality oils may contain contaminants or synthetic additives.

★Herbal remedies particularly garlic, hawthorn berries, coenzyme Q10, and fish oil, have proven benefits for heart health. Garlic acts as a natural vasodilator, helping to widen arteries and reduce blood clot formation; hawthorn berries improve heart contractility and blood flow; Coenzyme Q10 enhances the production of energy within the cells, contributing to improved heart function; and fish oil contains Omega-3 fatty acids, which help maintain proper heart rhythm and prevent plaque buildup in artery walls. Consulting a knowledgeable healthcare practitioner will ensure you choose appropriate dosages based on individual needs.

★Acupuncture is an ancient healing art rooted in Traditional Chinese Medicine. Practitioners insert fine needles at precise points on the body to correct imbalances in vital life energies. Research suggests that acupuncture can help regulate heart rate, improve blood pressure, and alleviate symptoms associated with angina (chest pain). This non-invasive treatment carries minimal side effects, making it a safe option for individuals seeking alternatives to conventional treatments.

★ Massage therapy offers numerous benefits for

heart health through its ability to relax muscles, improve circulation, and release tense muscles around the heart. Specific massage techniques like myofascial release, trigger point therapy, or Swedish massage can address muscular imbalances and encourage better posture – both critical components of maintaining a healthy circulatory system.

★Exercise regularly While not strictly "alternative," incorporating regular physical activity into your lifestyle is crucial for optimizing heart health. The American Heart Association recommends at least 150 minutes per week of moderate intensity aerobic activities or 75 minutes per week of vigorous aerobic exercises combined with muscle strengthening activities two days a week. Choose enjoyable activities such as walking, cycling, swimming, gardening, or dancing to keep your heart active and strong.

★Lastly, consider exploring the benefits of **Tai Chi and Qigong.** These traditional Chinese practices involve slow, deliberate movements coordinated with breath control and focused intention. Tai Chi is often described as 'meditation in motion,' providing both cardiovascular workout and stress relief. By practicing Tai Chi and Qigong consistently, you can develop greater awareness, resilience, and inner peace while fortifying your heart and entire being.

Each chapter presented unique strategies for

managing stress, supporting heart functions, preventing illnesses, and improving overall wellbeing. It's essential to remember that no single approach works best for everyone. Instead, integrating multiple evidence-based methods tailored to individual preferences and circumstances can yield remarkable results.

By embracing a multidimensional perspective on heart health, we empower ourselves with the knowledge and tools necessary to foster a stronger, healthier heart. Together, let us embark upon this journey towards Heart Harmony – enriching our lives through balanced choices and compassionate self-care. May the lessons learned here inspire hope, healing, and happiness as we move forward with courage and determination.

Take the first step today – explore, experiment, and embrace these alternative therapies. Your heart, mind, and soul will thank you!